Mind Your Healing!

How To Get Healing Out Of The Way So That You Can Step Into Other Dimensions Of Your Life

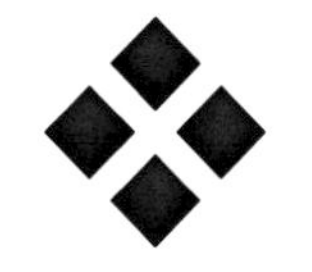

DR. ALBERT M. KIM ND
A NATUROPATHIC PHYSICIAN

Mind Your Healing! How To Get Healing Out of the Way
So That You Can Step Into Other Dimensions of Your Life

Copyright © 2012 Albert M. Kim
All Rights Reserved.
Unauthorized duplication or distribution is strictly prohibited.

ISBN 10: 0983169896
ISBN 13: 978-0-9831698-9-5

The purpose of this book is to educate and entertain. The author and/or publisher do not guarantee that anyone using these techniques, suggestions, tips, ideas or strategies will meet with success. The author and/or publisher shall have neither liability nor responsibility to anyone with respect to any loss or damage caused, or alleged to be caused, directly or indirectly by the information contained in this book.

Published by: Expert Author Publishing
http://expertauthorpublishing.com

Canadian Address:
1265 Charter Hill Drive
Coquitlam, BC, V3E 1P1

US Address:
1300 Boblett Street
Unit A-218
Blaine, WA 98230

Table of Contents

Foreword	7
Introduction	12
Where are the heroes?	16
You have the power to make miracles happen	19
Self-healing is self-evident	21
The healing power is within you	24
The secret key that unlocks all healing	25
Friendship can trigger a healing response	27
The wise have one eye on the cause, and the other eye on the result	31
The road to health is determined by you	33
The five healing thoughts	35
Your doctor is not a healer, but the best ***assistant*** to the healer	36
Best treatments establish the conditions for healing to take place	38
Return to your center	41
A lesson from a pair of compasses	42
Reduce the sensory pollutions	44
The breakthrough insights are in the realm of the sixth sense	49
Actions turn an insight into a reality	53
The top ten killers are heavily influenced by one's lifestyle	55
There is a race between healing and injury	58
Joint injuries can be cured if treated early	60
Health and fitness are two different things	63
The forgotten ingredients for an extraordinary life	66
Wisdom—the first ingredient for an extraordinary life	68
Compassion—the second ingredient for an extraordinary life	71
Courage—the third ingredient of an extraordinary life	74
A mature person masters all three virtues	77
An enlightened person is someone who has gone back to become a child, ***tzu***	78
Humans are capable of continued growth	83

A life truly worth living is worth recording 84
To increase the mind power, one has to ***decrease*** the number of thoughts 85
Helping children develop their three virtues 87
Unresolving stress is the health enemy number one 89
Everything is made twice: once in mind, and then in form 91
We are One 93
Ultimately, our problem will be a problem of time—the lack of it 95
Existentialism 98
You already have the most important things 100
You have a sophisticated healing system 104
The misunderstood story of cholesterol 107
Why it is harmful to blindly lower cholesterol 111
The misunderstood story of osteoporosis 116
Like any intelligent system, your body demands respect 120
As diseases deeply root, effective treatments become more invasive 121
Your potential life span is 150 years 122
Most of us are born with a great constitution for health 124
Find a doctor who knows your health condition well 126
Focus on things that a few things that truly matter 128
Nutrients are the building blocks of your body 130
Eating the Small COW diet 132
Further exploration into plant toxins 136
Eating well 142
Humanity began cooking 1.9 million years ago 143
The circulatory system and the lymphatic system 145
Improving the delivery of nutrients into cells through muscle contraction 146
Exercising the power of faith 149
The miller, his son and the donkey 151
Fear paralyzes 154
Have fewer thoughts 156
Your empowering vision keeps you focused 158
Brief Reflection on Maps 160
Two Brothers 161

Quality of life through the depth of love 163
Evolution of human consciousness 166
Enlightenment in a coin 169
Four ways to overcome stress 173
Imagine 174
Endnotes 176

Foreword

Dr. Habib Sadeghi DO

The world has changed more in the last thirty years than it has in the previous hundred. If you are over 40, chances are that you have far more in common with your grandparents' simpler lifestyle than your own children's. Everything is moving faster. People want what they want, know exactly how they want it, and they want it *now*. Technological advancements in every facet of life from food service to personal communication have made instant gratification more than just a reality. It has made instant gratification a *necessity*. If we expect to keep up with a world that is moving at a breakneck pace, we have to keep increasing the speed of our own treadmill.

Convenience, however, has its price. As we have become overly dependent on others, and especially on our personal communication devices to do more for us, we have become *less*. I cannot tell you how many people I run into who cannot memorize a seven-digit phone number that has been recited to them, so they need to have their cell phone in hand to program it immediately. In the near future, I wonder how many will remember how to make pierogies from scratch, recite an inspiring poem by heart, or perform basic math in their mind.

Such activities themselves do not carry as much weight as the rather unconscious cognitive processes that lie beneath such performances. Every time we master a new skill, every time we memorize a new song or a poem, every time we perform simple calculations in our own mind—we are indeed *rewiring* our neural network. We are *restructuring* our brains to become accustomed to a whole new way of thinking…and *being.*

Thus it is an irony that the technological gadgets that have made instant connection with someone a continent away into a reality have also disconnected us from each other in a very fundamental, visceral and spiritual way. Just walk into a coffee shop and you would be surprised to see how less and less common it is to catch two people actually having coffee and *talking* to each other, instead of the many lone visitors, sitting by themselves, texting, wearing headphones or staring into their laptop screens.

In a world that is moving dreadfully fast, convenience has cost us dearly. We have traded *mindfulness* for *multi-tasking*; *intuition* for *automation.* It seems that as our virtual connections become stronger, our spiritual connections to each other and ourselves become weaker. As this continues, we have become less present in the now, and less present "in our bodies." Without this vital interface between mind and body, it is simply impossible to know our true state of health at any given time.

Our *Mind* and *Body* are not "talking" to each other. If you examine the wave of new and emerging chronic diseases that have appeared over the last several decades, you will find that they are juxtaposed almost perfectly with the dawn of the so-called Information Age. Allowing ourselves to be entangled by the information that drives the world keeps us stuck "in form." However, if we *choose* to look inward and connect with that which inspires us, we remain "in spirit".

It's no coincidence that as disease rates have climbed, the profit margins of the pharmaceutical corporations have sky-rocketed. While I'm not excusing the subversive marketing tactics of "big pharma," I see an increasing number of patients who are disconnected from their own bodies. As such, they have learned to *do less for themselves* and have *abdicated 100%* of the responsibility of their healthcare to their doctors, drugs, gadgets, and others—anything that is *outside* of themselves.

To make it worse, some of today's patients do not desire to invest any time or energy into overcoming their own illnesses. It is as though their illness is someone else's job to "fix me." Of course, it is because it is easier to take a pill to numb the symptoms rather than dealing with the root cause of the problem that is causing the constellation of symptoms. That is why many patients arrive at the doctor's office in the *end stages* of disease—many times because they were completely unaware of what was happening within their own bodies for many years.

This is not to place blame on patients, but to display how we have all become *unplugged* from our *innate healing power* and how we have handed our wellness over to those whose motives may lie elsewhere.

In his exciting new book, *Mind Your Healing,* my esteemed colleague, Dr. Albert M. Kim explains that all the healing power you will ever need to "live with renewed vitality" is within you. That is not a spiritual euphemism or a feel-good phrase. Dr. Kim details in a clear and concise way how you can get off the stress-fueled "hamster wheel" and initiate your own healing. His research into all the great spiritual traditions of the world will reveal to you the common thread that runs through all of them with regard to healing—*When we can set a powerful intention and remain focused on it while simultaneously anchoring our attention in every present moment from a trusting place within ourselves, healing happens naturally.*

His simple and practical principles are as enlightening as they are empowering. They will put your healthcare back where it should be, in your own hands. This is because you are the expert in YOU. Dr. Kim shows you how to unplug from what is draining you, and plug back in to your higher awareness.

Healing is not a magic trick. It is not even a miracle. It is as common to human beings as breathing. We have just lost our connection with this innate gift so much that when healing does occur, we call it *astonishing*, *magical*, and *miraculous*! In fact, the opposite is true. The miracle is that we are surviving as well as we are with all the suppressing of our healing tendencies within us and by making unhealthy lifestyle choices. Dr. Kim takes the mystery out of healing, and shows you that you do not have to be a guru or a saint to create miraculous healing in your life right now.

Health is an intimate part of life, and our quality of life is determined by the choices we make. That is all life really is—a single choice that leads to the next choice and so on. When we make smarter choices, our life and health improve exponentially. When we remain present and connected to ourselves, we naturally choose the path that leads to health and healing. However, we have to make that first choice. Selecting this book is that first choice on your healing journey. The next will be to implement Dr. Kim's valuable knowledge. When you do, you'll see that the power to accomplish anything you desire, not just your health goals, that has been beyond your reach. You are the biggest secret that you have been seeking.

Glinda the good witch in Frank L. Baum's classic *The Wizard of Oz* gives us a great example of the immense power we possess, but fail to see. At the end of her arduous journey, Dorothy begs the good witch to send her back home. Glinda replies that Dorothy *always* had the power to send herself back home at any time she chose through the power in the magical shoes she wore along her entire adventure. So my dear friends, you have the same power within in you. Enjoy awakening to your own magnificence and the journey that will lead you back to the savior that you have been searching for all along…You!

Dr. Habib Sadeghi DO
Be Hive of Healing
Los Angeles, California
April 2012

Introduction

Dr. Timothy Brown DC, ND

There is a saying that "young souls" on this planet are interested in *receiving* while "older souls" are interested in *giving*.

As these older souls continue to grow, they enthusiastically share with the world the precious gems of wisdom that they have collected—be it person to person, or in other ways, such as writing a book that can reach out to the whole world.

In this regard, Dr. Albert Kim is an old soul. He has a relentless passion for learning the principles of life, mastering them, and sharing his accumulated gems of wisdom with the rest of the world.

You are holding that very book, entirely made up of those *gems of wisdom*.

For example, as you read the book, you will see that there are four primary factors in life that create either *freedom* or *stress* depending on their relationship to us. When decisions are made, these are also the four primary factors that shape our decision-making. These four primary factors are Career, Relationship, Health and Wealth.

In a "freedom" cycle these factors are expansive and the *sense of freedom* comes from having the *mastery* over these areas. Career flows effortlessly. Relationships provide solid network to build further love and prosperity. Health provides the ready energy for one to take effective action steps. Abundant wealth reserve keeps one in the *thriving* mode.

In converse, when these factors are *compressed* in the "stress" cycle—they push on us to feel the *stress* of career hardships, feelings of isolation and disconnect in life, limited energy coming from an unreliable body, and the little wealth reserve that dries up too quickly. These keep one in the perpetual *survival* mode.

Dr. Kim's book, *Mind Your Healing!* focuses on the principles of *mastery in healing*. Healing is the most important aspect of the four primary factors in life. Mastery of health requires the integrated functioning between the Body, Mind and Spirit. Without proper relationship between these three aspects of Being, there exists an interference with one's ability to carry on functioning, and later on, tap into the other higher "dimensions" of life.

As doctors we see the *effects* of injuries, such as the resulting emotional and mental traumas, toxicity and infections. These further contribute to patients choosing unhealthy lifestyles, and consequently their inability to overcome their ill circumstances. As doctors, we also witness the miraculous and gratifying results when patients "untangle" and *free* themselves from the *obstacles to healing!*

Dr. Kim has studied and searched for the precious but often hidden *principles of healing* that have made a profound difference when applied in the *lives of his patients*.

As you read this book—each chapter being short and succinct—I encourage you to reflect on the principles and the wisdom behind the writing. Each chapter is a timeless principle of life itself, and you may find that these principles are *familiar* to you in two ways. Firstly, these principles are found in the *wisdom writings of the ages*—both Western and Eastern. Secondly, these may be *your own stories of your heroic journey in this life*.

As you read each chapter, contemplate on an area of your life. May you find inspiration to incorporate these precious principles into massive action steps, so that you too can "... get healing out of the way, so that you can step into *other* dimensions of your life."

Dr. Timothy Brown DC, ND

Once you get healing out of the way,
You step into other dimensions of your life.

Once you solve the health problem,
The time and energy will avail themselves to you,
For you to work on other meaningful projects.

For that reason alone,
Healing is a worthwhile objective.

With love and light,
Albert M. Kim ND

Where are the heroes?

With every discouraging news reported—of death, murder, and diseases—there are thousands of unreported heart-warming events. That is why it is so encouraging to see what a group of bystanders did in Logan, Utah on September 13, 2011 when a motorcyclist became trapped under a burning car. People rushed over to save the 21-year-old motorcyclist, Brandon Wright, from a certain death.[1]

The motorcycle burned up ferociously. Judging by the flames, the gas cap must have come loose, and the gasoline caught fire. A man wearing blue-green shirt tried to lift the car by himself, but couldn't. Then a construction worker came and tried to lift the car. He couldn't. Then four others joined, including a lady, to lift the car. However, six wasn't enough to lift the car. The lady got on her belly to see how the motorcyclist was doing under the car that was burning furiously. She pointed to everyone that the motorcyclist was still there, pinned under the car.

More people joined in, about eight altogether. They tried lifting again, and they succeeded in lifting the car to about 40 degrees, and a construction worker grabbed hold of the motorcyclist's right ankle and pulled him out to safety. The motorcyclist survived, and he later says in the hospital bed that he should have died three times—when he first hit the concrete without a helmet on, when he collided with the car, and when the car burst into flames[2].

According to Joseph Campbell, a hero is an ordinary person, leading an ordinary life. Then one day, the hero is called to an adventure. The hero refuses to heed it. But eventually something pushes the hero to accept the call. When the hero is committed; magical tools, mentors and supporters appear to arm, inspire and assist the hero. After all, the hero has to cross the river of boiling lava and face the fire-breathing dragon. The Universe never sends the hero unprepared for the challenges. In such a way, the hero leaves behind the known limits of his world, and crosses into the unknown land of adventure. There, the hero faces the ultimate nemesis, the dragon, slays the dragon, and brings home the treasures. When he returns home, the town is the same, but he is a changed person.

A hero is not born. A hero is made. A hero starts out as an ordinary person. An opportunity knocks. When you respond to the call, you have become a hero.

Find a mirror and look at yourself reflected on it. Look into those eyes *looking* right back. What you see in the mirror are the eyes of the hero looking back. *You* are the hero that your community has been seeking. You are the hero that you have been seeking.

The Lord said to Moses, "Why are you crying out to Me?"
Exodus 14:15.

You have the power to make miracles happen

One of the most insightful events in the Bible occurs when Moses divides the Red Sea. The Pharaoh's evil army was charging at the people of Israel—with the intent to slaughter everyone. The dividing of the Red Sea created a safe passage for the people of Israel to cross the sea and escape the Pharaoh's evil army.

The dividing of the Red Sea itself is a miracle, but there is an even greater miracle hidden within. It is not the act of bending the *elements*. Rather it is the bending of people's *hearts* that is the true miracle in that story. God forever changed the way Moses saw how life works. Let's explore further.

When the people of Israel were camping by the Red Sea, the army of the Pharaoh charged at them with the order to slaughter them. The people of Israel knew that they were facing a certain death. They began blaming Moses for their terrible fate. They cried out to Moses, "Is it because there were no graves in Egypt that you have taken us away to die in the wilderness?" Moses tried to rekindle the Israelite's faith in God and spoke,

"Do not fear... The Lord will fight for you."

Upon hearing this, God spoke to Moses,

"Why are you crying out to Me?"

God continued,

"Lift up your staff and stretch out your hand over the sea and divide it."

God was telling Moses not to rely on Him or anyone else, because Moses himself has *the ability* to make miracles happen. All he had to do is to command. For Moses to divide the sea, all he needed to do was to *command* the sea to do so!

It would have been a miracle if God split the sea *for* Moses. But even *greater* miracle happened when Moses learned that he could, too, split the sea. In the most desperate moment of all times, Moses connected with God. God was gentle enough to guide him to his awakening. He understood God. That was when Moses understood the nature of the universe.

Just like Moses, *you have the power to make miracles happen.*

Self-healing is self-evident

There is a secret that everyone can benefit by knowing it, but scarcely anyone seems to know. It is a secret *not* because someone had hidden it. In fact, it is as obvious as the sun in the sky. It is a secret simply because people have *become* unaware of it. What is this secret?

It is your ability to self-heal.

Self-healing is self-evident. It is obvious. It is so obvious that we often throw it out of our mind. Consider what happens when you get a little cut on your finger. It heals. Your body is capable of self-healing. If it can heal a cut, it can heal your other ailments too.

It is *not* a doctor who has the power to heal you. It is *you* who does the healing. A doctor performs a treatment. But it is you who does the healing. Without a self-healing ability, no treatment would ever work. Did you know that there are no treatments in the whole world that can heal a cut made on a piece of steak. A treatment does not heal, and is never meant to heal. It merely functions to assist your healing.

If there is one statement that summarizes this entire book, it is this. ***You are the Healer that you seek.*** You are the key to healing your health challenges.

But you say that you had the same diabetic ulcer on your shin for the past several years, that you had terrible migraine headaches for the past many years, or that you had high blood pressure for the past many more years! So how can you be a healer when you have all these illnesses, which are not healing, you ask.

You see, when an injury does not heal, it isn't because you don't have the *ability* to heal. You have the perfect healing mechanism within you.

However, there are things that can impede this healing mechanism, which prevents it from working properly. A skilful gardener knows that the seeds sown in the garden cannot grow if too many things impede their growth.

This is the reason why you need a doctor—to help you *remove* the obstacles to your healing. A doctor's role is to support your healing.

A doctor does the treating. But YOU do the healing.

Become the light to yourself
In a world that is becoming increasingly dark.
Jiddu Krishnamurti

The healing power is within you

Illness is an undeniable certainty in life.
Everyone will become ill at one time or another.

Susan had been getting comments from her friends whether she was trying to get tanned lately. Back at home, she looked at her face in the mirror, and found that her face did, in fact, looked remarkably dark, but not gorgeous sun-kissed dark. Her skin was dull and lifeless. She thought it was strange. One of her uncles was a doctor and she went to see him about her condition. Her uncle decided to do a few tests. Within a few days, she found herself lying in a hospital bed with diagnosis of malignant liver cancer. "What just happened?" she asked herself.

That was over ten years ago, and Susan is OK now. She is in remission, with no signs of cancer. She was one of those few lucky outliers who have miraculously recovered from an aggressive form of cancer. Some people, like Susan, heal remarkably. Why is this so?

The secret key that unlocks all healing

Sufferings are the taxes of life.
Everyone pays.
But some pay too much.

An illness can go on for months, and sometimes stretches into years. It is exhausting, and people lose their spirit. They feel trapped in an unpleasant condition that they are not able to shake loose from the illness and be free. As a result they become irritable and exhausted, and they are easily triggered into anger and depression.

But there is a way out of an illness. There is a key that unlocks all healing. This key is the potent power that exists in every individual.

The good news is that the potent power is working in everyone—including in *you*. All you have to do is for you to *access* to this great power of healing mechanism. *Every individual has the power to self-heal.* This formidable power is inherent in everyone.

This *healing mechanism* works all the time from one's birth to death. In fact, one dies when this force no longer can conquer the injuries inflicted on the body.

It is this healing mechanism that is pumping your heart. It is this force that is making you breathe when you are asleep. It is this healing mechanism that digests the food that you have eaten. It is this force that repairs the injuries that you have.

The seventy-five trillion cells in one's body are working in perfect coordination to maintain one's life—to allow one to see, hear, feel, smell, taste, think, digest and sweat. A person cannot do this consciously. It is done at the unconscious level.

There is the healing mechanism within every individual who is alive, and it looks after all the vital functions of life. It is a miracle when one considers what must be coordinated so perfectly in order to keep one alive and functioning.

This great force of healing mechanism has been observed in many cultures. It goes by different names in different cultures, but they all refer to the same observation.

Different traditions called it by different names. In the ancient Chinese healing tradition, this great force is called *Qi* (pronounced "chi"). The ancient Greeks called it *Pneuma.* The ancient Hindus called it *Prana.* In classical Hippocratic medicine, it is called *nosos feisis iatree* in Greek. In Latin, it is called *vis medicatrix naturae*, translated into English, "the power that heals *on its own*[3]." The healing mechanism is perhaps the most essential aspect of one's life, yet it remains unrecognized in the majority of the population.

Friendship can trigger a healing response

A lover brings heaven and hell,
But a friend brings only heaven.

Susan left the hospital to die at home. The hospital informed her that she had three months to live. The last thing she wanted to do was to die in an unfamiliar, sterile environment. At home she had her comfortable couch, her warm bed, her favorite books, and her dining set that she admires when she has her meals. Most of all, she wanted to die in her own familiar environment in peace.

Her husband had abandoned her some years ago, and fortunately they didn't have any children to worry about. Her parents had passed on, and all she had were her pesky relatives who always wanted *something* from her—either in the form of money, her energy or her time—and often all of them. None of those resources could she spare now.

When she came home, she immediately picked up the phone and began calling everyone that she is going away on a trip for a year. This was a tactic to keep people away. But Susan had a friend, Mary, who cared about her dearly, so she told Mary the truth. Susan asked Mary a favor. She asked Mary whether she could help out by bringing her some groceries and check her mailbox while she was making the transition from Earth to the "the other world." Mary agreed with tears.

However, it turned out that Mary was not such a compliant helper. Mary would bring Susan all kinds of supplements and herbs, and made sure Susan took them. Susan didn't believe that her condition was curable, and she had refused initially. But Mary wouldn't give in. So, *Susan* gave in. Susan began taking them, but most of the pills she would simply vomit out. Susan finally said that she couldn't hold them down, so she will no longer take any pills.

Mary stopped offering anything for a couple of days. Then, she brought in the acai juice. Mary reasoned that if pills were too hard to swallow, juice would be fine. Susan knew how stubborn Mary could get. So to preserve the *peace*, she began taking it. But it was only for a few days. Susan lost the desire to continue on this way. She felt no one cared for her. And she cared for no one. "What's the point of living in a world without love?" she asked.

She decided to "will" herself to die, and she was making one last phone call. It was to the only person who ever showed any true friendship—Mary. On the phone, she told Mary that she stopped taking the acai juice, and she was going to let it all go. That was when Mary blurted out something that shook up her soul. Mary said that she was never popular like Susan was, and she never had any other friends. Susan was the only friend she's got. Mary said that she could live without a lover, but she couldn't live without a friend.

Susan had never heard anything like that before. But she couldn't agree more. All this time, thick and thin, joyous and painful, she could deal with the losses of many things—including her own husband with relative composure and grace, but she couldn't have lived without the friendship that Mary offered. Susan gave in again to Mary. Susan began to take the acai juice faithfully.

One day, Susan felt like she wanted to throw up. She hurried to the bathroom, and began vomiting into the toilet bowl. She was surprised by the beet-red vomit. It was all bloody. She never had bloody vomit before. After rinsing her mouth, she looked at herself in the bathroom mirror, and told herself that the time was up. She was most likely going to die now. On her way back to her favorite couch, she collapsed on the floor, and lost consciousness.

When she regained her consciousness, she wasn't sure whether she was dead or alive. Something was different. Normally, her body would be heavy and achy, but the body felt light and pain free. So she thought that she was probably dead. She stood up and opened the window. It was a warm, sunny, beautiful day outside. She put on her jacket and went out for a walk. She actually could walk for several minutes without any discomfort. She initiated a small chat with a stranger, and decided that she must be still alive. Her energy, along with appetite and mood came back. Since that day, she has been in remission from her cancer.

So what is the secret of her success in beating her cancer?

To this date, she believes it was the acai berry juice. She tells me that I should be drinking it on a daily basis to prevent all cancers.

Acai juice probably helped. However, I don't believe for a single moment that acai or any physical remedy has the power to cure terminal cancers. A physical ailment needs a higher vibration than itself for the healing to take place.

So what triggered healing in Susan?

In my humble opinion, it was the *friendship*—the friendship that Mary offered to Susan. The high vibration of pure friendship raised Susan's emotional energy. With the increase in energy, she brought all her cells back into focus to give life another chance.

The wise have one eye on the cause, and the other eye on the result

All great heroes have one thing in common. They have one eye on the Great Cause and the other eye locked on the Great Result. The Great Cause is the now; and the Great Result is the goal well achieved.

People instinctively become concerned with the *results*, at the expense of their concern for the *causes*. They become *hyperopic*—far-sighted, and can't see the opportunities that are constantly passing by. When people suffer from an illness, they look for ways to bring an end to the symptoms—symptoms such as fever and pain. All energy is put to resolve the symptoms, but at the cost of treating the cause.

It is common to see a patient with hypertension (high blood pressure) to be medicated with purely symptomatic medications such as beta-blockers, ACE inhibitors, thiazide water pills and calcium channel blockers. When their blood pressure is suppressed to reduced numbers, everyone seems to find satisfaction in this suppressive therapy and stops searching for the cause. The purpose of symptomatic relief is to buy time—so that one can heal the illness with the least amount of suffering. But no one should make the mistake of taking the symptomatic control as the cure itself.

Some people become obsessed with the causes, and become myopic or near-sighted. They neglect the feedback from the world, which can offer valuable insight for the navigation towards their Great Result.

Life can be compared to sailing through the vast seas. It requires a predetermined destination and the ability to ride the changing winds and currents. Although I am not personally a fan of warriors, Alexander the Great did great things, albeit terrible things. After all, he forcefully conquered half the world, killing a massive number of innocent men, women, seniors and children.

The legends say that his secret was his unique ability to have one eye set on the *Now,* and the other eye set on the *Future*. Alexander may have been a brutal warrior, but he was nonetheless great in achieving things that are commonly considered impossible.

In order to reach your great goals, have one eye steadfast on the result; while having the other eye on the now. Now is the only time you can make any changes. No one can even for a second visit the past or the future. That is why Now *is* the Cause that can incubate the future that you desire.

The road to health is determined by you

As people become concerned with their illnesses, they begin to think in terms of their ability to function while being ill. People believe that health determines what they can do and cannot do. They believe that health puts a limit to what they get to be, the work they can do, the lifestyle they can lead, the relationship that they can have, and the wealth they can achieve.

In a short term, health does somewhat determine what anyone can and cannot do. However, health—or the lack of it—is a condition. Every condition can be likened to a pile of mud that can be worked on and *shaped* into what the artist desires. In time, by working on the things that truly matter, all conditions can be made favorable. Since an individual can shape the conditions by working on them, in the long run, it is *the individual* who determines how healthy one gets to be.

In Korea, there is a saying, "*It is better to be wallowing in mud, than to be dead.*" When one finds himself in the worst possible set of conditions, there is still hope. By diligently working on the conditions, one can make tremendous changes within a year or two. On the other hand, when we are dead, the chapter is closed, and the book of life finished. No matter how terrible the conditions, it is still better to be alive, so that we can start walking towards our particular dreams.

The road to health is determined by *you.* It is you who has the power to allow health to blossom. This starts with a flash of an *insight* that reveals to the conscious mind what is possible.

Health affects us all. It cares not for your career, religion, culture, ethnicity, philosophy, sex, age or wealth. Health touches everyone. The problem is that people are *not* touching their health.

The five healing thoughts

1. I am a healer.
2. I am the *only* healer who can heal me.
3. I cannot heal anyone else.
4. I heal when the conditions are met.
5. I don't have the true personal power until I know how to meet those conditions.

Your doctor is not a healer, but the best *assistant* to the healer

In order to heal, you allow this healing force to express itself in its most potent state—just as a skilled farmer allows his crops to flourish by giving them the right conditions.

There are only two ways to accelerate healing. First is to strengthen the healing mechanism. The second is through removing the obstacles that get in the way of the healing mechanism.

The history has examples of famous healers. These include Jesus Christ, Gautama Buddha and St. Francis of Assisi. They were known to be able to heal the sick and the dying. They were healers, and they healed people.

However, an average person cannot heal someone else—unless he also happens to have reached the level of awareness of Jesus, Gautama or Francis who has ascended and found ways to reach out and manifest healing beyond self-healing.

But what about the doctors? Are not doctors healers?

A doctor being a healer is a myth and a misunderstanding. An ordinary doctor cannot heal. In fact, it is not even a duty of a doctor to heal.

Various doctors use different modalities of healing, but none of them can heal someone else. A doctor is an *assistant* to the healing mechanism, but not a healer. An analogy can be found in farming. A farmer does not have the special ability to make the crops grow. A farmer can only assist their growth. A farmer who cares for his crops provides the crops with appropriate fertilizers and removes harmful pests. A skilled doctor who cares for his patients provides the healing mechanism of that patient with whatever the patient needs in order to heal.

A doctor finds out what is missing in a patient with an illness by (1) taking inventory of the constellation of symptoms, and (2) deducing the cause of those symptoms. Then (3) the doctor provides the correct remedies that reduce the symptoms while eliminating the cause of the illness. The correct remedy may be setting the broken bones and then casting after the surgery. Then the doctor prescribes the bone building supplements and, later, a set of proper exercises to strengthen the bones.

Once the appropriate treatment is done, a doctor steps back and let Nature do her miracles. Hence the title physician [Latin *physica* "Natural Science," *–an* "one who practices."]

The title, physician in its original meaning symbolized *a person who observes Nature, studies Nature, and practices the Natural Science to help people heal.* A doctor and a healer are two separate entities. This idea has been emphasized by many influential thinkers, such as François-Marie Arouet (aka Voltaire). He once said, "A doctor entertains the patient while *Nature* heals the patient." Indeed this isn't so far from fact. A doctor *treats* a patient, but Nature *heals* the patient.

Everyone is a healer. But the healing ability is limited to self-healing. Only the ones who have reached a certain level of awakening can heal someone else.

Best treatments establish the conditions for healing to take place

An adept gardener considers carefully whether the plants are getting too much water or too little water, too much sunshine or too little sunshine. Too *much* or too *little* of what is needed can impede health of the plants. When the gardener finds that the lawn yellowing and burning up, he turns on the sprinklers to rehydrate them. If the plants are failing to thrive, the gardener may add the appropriate fertilizers to help the plants to thrive.

A doctor's mission is to help you return to health. But he cannot do this directly. He helps you by removing the obstacles to healing. Your doctor's role is to assist you in removing the obstacles to healing, and deliver the right conditions for healing to take place. A doctor treats while the patient heals himself.

A skilful doctor is, therefore, a skilful detective. He is a Sherlock Holmes solving the mystery of *whodunit*. A skilful detective doctor pieces together all the correct clues and picks out the *cause* of the problem. The doctor then provides the body with the correct remedies, and healing takes place.

For example, the body may not be healing because it is in need of some nutrients.

What is a nutrient?

Whichever part of your body you touch, nutrients make up

those cells and tissues. In other words, nutrients are the *building blocks* of your body.

If the body is lacking the needed nutrients, the body cannot heal—just as you cannot complete a construction of an impressive architectural structure when you are lacking the needed building blocks. The healing power inherent in people cannot repair the body without the necessary nutrients.

Another remedy may be resting. The body cannot endure the prolonged periods of activity without resting. It is because resting provides a timeout from further injuries. Resting and sleeping provide moments of peace from the stressors of life. During resting, the body redirects the vital energy and nutrients to produce the healing components needed for healing—such as the hormones, enzymes and cells from the nutrient building blocks.

The inherent healing power needs the support from both individuals and the experienced doctors. Supporting your inherent healing mechanism is truly the only way to heal injuries and illnesses. This inherent healing power is also what is needed to maintain the best health, so that the body remains *reliable*.

Here is a crucial question that people should ask. Why bother having a healthy and reliable body?

In one sense, a healthy reliable body is free of chronic pain and suffering. That would be some of the convincing reasons to be healthy, but not all of the reasons.

In a larger sense, a healthy and reliable body is required as a firm foundation. Health is the firm foundation on top of which everything great that one desires to create on Earth can stand.

The body has to be relatively pain-free and full of Qi before there is enough peace of mind and the mental horsepower to tap into one's *higher purposes* on Earth. Then, one can express the unique gifts and talents for the world that he is a part of. *You can heal because you are powerful beyond measure.*

Dr. Wayne Dyer, the author of Wisdom of Ages, once called the universe—a "uni-verse." He used the word "Uni" to mean *one*, and the word "verse" to suggest a *song*. If the universe is just One Grand Song, you are a segment of musical notes that make up the Grand Song.

Your very *Being* with all your unique gifts and talents are the notes that are needed to complete the "uni-verse." In other words, without you, the Great Song of the universe would be incomplete.

Provide the body with what the healing mechanism needs to heal. This is the quickest path to healing.

Return to your center

What a different story people would have to tell
if they would adopt a definite purpose and stand
by that purpose until it had time to become an
all-consuming purpose.
Napoleon Hill (Law of Success)

To be centered one has to have a point of reference—a starting point. The starting point of one's actions is a decision. The word, *decide* is made up of two components: *de* meaning "off" and *cidere* meaning "to cut." *Decide* literally means to "cut off" the ends, the non-priorities of your life. To be decisive about health, one has to sort out what *is* and *is not* essential for manifesting a solid state of health.

A powerful form of decision is declaration. A declaration is one's *official decision* clearly stated to the *public*. It will clearly state one's decision in black and white. A declaration comes from a person who has done the soul searching and resurfaced to the world with a firm grasp of one's resolution. Such declaration can serve as the spark that starts up the engine of one's health. A well-constructed declaration can inject certainty into one's actions that follow. An action, which is supported by certainty, matures into a set of behaviors that lead one to manifesting. That is how one becomes centered.

A lesson from a pair of compasses

Gnōthi sauton — "Know Thyself"

Try drawing a circle with a pencil. The circle that is drawn turns out, at best to be a *wiggly* circle. But one pulls out a pair of compasses, and he can begin drawing perfect circles every time!

What makes a pair of compasses so capable of drawing perfect circles time after time is in its mechanism. A pair of compasses has two arms—one is the firmly anchored inner arm onto which the instrument pivots around, and the moving outer arm that draws the circle. It is because of the anchoring arm the instrument can draw perfect circles.

The analogy stands for our *decision* and *behavior* as the anchoring arm and the drawing arm. The anchoring arm is the decision, and the drawing arm is the behavior that flows out *naturally* as a result of that firm decision.

Just as the pair of compasses needs the anchoring arm, your whole Being needs to know your decision. A firm decision creates a solid manifestation. A wobbly decision creates a wobbly manifestation. Someone who has not decided cannot be said to be well anchored, and thus *wobbles* in his daily life. He will consequently lack the effective behaviors that lead to the massive fruition.

An old Buddhist saying goes, there is *a time for meditation and a time for action.*

After getting your intent clarified into a laser-sharp decision, it is time for your action. Action is crucial for success. A farmer cannot just sow the seeds and then leave the fields abandoned. Cultivation is needed to keep the noxious weeds and the harmful insects away from the young and fragile crops.

Success is a consequence of a firm decision *and* clear actions that follow—not the mere decision alone. Clear actions follow a firm decision like the shadow that follows the object. Such actions should have one vector—the direction and magnitude of the force of actions point to the manifestation of the decided goal. These actions should be self-evident to any rational observer. These actions thus lead to an eventual success—in this case, overcoming illnesses, and achieving health.

So decide to be healthy. Once decided, your intent will become clearer, so that your actions can begin to align themselves, just as how a circle is drawn with a pair of compasses—effortlessly and perfectly!

Reduce the sensory pollutions

Five senses may be adequate for maintaining the *status quo*, but insights belong to the realm of the *sixth sense*. The sixth senses are needed to make a magnificent transformation. Let's first explore the world of the five senses.

Your sense of sight, hearing, touch, smell and taste comprise the five senses. These are known in psychology as visual, auditory, kinesthetic, olfactory and gustatory senses. These five senses can be collectively called *vakog*, after taking the initials of each word.

These five senses—visual (seeing), auditory (hearing), kinesthetic (sensation of touch), olfactory (smelling), and gustatory (taste)—are supposed to provide the accurate data about the world around us. Fifty thousand years ago, it might have served us adequately, but now the humanity has the need for a source of information that is beyond the five senses.

The modern world has flooded the humanity with excessive levels of sensual stimulation, and many are not useful, many are negative, and some are even false. Instead of giving humanity some accurate feedback of the surrounding world as *per* its design, the five senses have come to serve as the shell of an egg that incubates within the illusions about life—blocking humanity from clarity of emotion, mind and spirit.

The sight pollution. Take an example of watching a beer commercial on TV. One beer commercial tried to paint a picture in the audience that the use of their beer transformed a lonely individual into a popular icon figure. You just saw with your own eyes how a lonely individual has transformed himself into a popular icon. So it certainly isn't a figment of your imagination. But you know this commercial is false.

There are no studies that show that alcohol makes an individual socially desirable. In fact, it makes the person much, *much less* desirable in many ways—the stench of alcohol on one's breath and clothing, the drunken behavior, and the loss of reasoning capacity, just to name a few—will get oneself an isolation chamber until he sobers up.

Newspapers tend to select negative events to report, and skip through the positive stories that happen in our society. They obsess over the shocking events, such as murders, rape, wars and other forms of mental and emotional violence. For example, the headlines of today's paper reads like this: "woman offered to pay hitmen $20,000 to kill her husband." "Two dead, two injured after SUV collides with tractor trailer." "More storms expected this week" and so on. These negative stories jar one's nerves. John Kehoe, the best-selling author of *Mind Power* says that with every negative event reported, there are hundreds of heart-warming positive events that take place around us all the time that go unreported.

Just a few days ago, I was standing at an intersection finishing up typing a short email message to a patient using my iPhone when I heard a "click" of someone pressing the walk button for the pedestrian light. I looked around and I saw a man walking away, pushing a baby cart. He had pushed the walk button for me because he saw me busy typing. Since he wasn't crossing the street, he pushed the button for the convenience of someone he didn't know. What he did warmed my heart and put a smile on my face. This was not because he did something for *me* personally, but because he showed *kindness* for a total stranger. These are the angels who glue the community together in harmony. Such events happen all the time, but go unnoticed. This is another reason why relying solely on newspapers for the world's events can skew one's perception of the reality of the world.

I once watched a movie where power tools gain evil consciousness of their own, and attempted to take over the world. They attacked any human being that got in their way in the most horrifying manner. I was *so relieved* when the movie was finally over, and pondered on the usefulness of such genre. I couldn't find any, perhaps other than to be careful with power tools, and perhaps a growing desire to stop watching movies altogether.

Startling visual stimulations constantly bombard us. I was out for my evening walk, and I just couldn't look away from the rapid flickering giant flat screen TV in someone's living room—all the way across the street. From a distance, I could see something that the viewer may not have noticed. Every fraction of a second, the scene changed rapidly. It was like someone kept flicking on and off the light switch. Each time I tried to look away, my attention kept going back to the TV. From a distance, the scenes appeared quite jerky to my eyes—and even when they were supposed to be still something about them kept flickering. This maybe a clever trick by the television industry to grab someone's attention. In biology, we learn that animals, including humans are attracted to sudden movements. This powerful biological predisposition is a reason why an ADHD child tends to sit through a TV show, but not able to sit through a classroom lecture.

The sound pollution. Then there are the noises that seem to be everywhere and anywhere. The *wailing* sirens of ambulances and fire trucks that cut through the silence of the night. The rumbling motorcycle exhaust sounds that wake up the neighborhood in the deep of the night. The neighbor's child practicing his new drum set down the block. The barking dog because the owner has left it alone. The "thin-skinned" car alarm that seems to go off whaling at 100 decibels whenever a gentle gust of wind blows by.

The excess kinesthetic stimulation. Then there is the excessive stimulation of the sensation of touch. The things we touch seem more and more artificial. They are no longer made up of grasses and the trees, but plastics and metals. There is less and less of the raindrops and sunshine on our skin, and more and more of the cold, flickering fluorescent lights and concrete walls surrounding us in our homes and offices.

The aches and pains attack our joints, instead of the sensation of joy and vigor coursing through the veins. The fast foods high in animal fats and trans fats have finally resulted in a culture where physical pain has become the norm. To add to the insult, people are working excessively. I personally know several people in a crippling physical condition who still work over 60 hours a week simply because without them, their company would have to file for bankruptcy and layoff many skilled workers. Many modern people live with pain as the norm.

The olfactory pollution. How about the overwhelming fragrances found in perfumes that people wear and products that we personally use on a daily basis?

Very recently I was in an elevator with a couple who seemed to have *bathed* in perfumes and aftershave lotion. I could feel my bronchi closing up to prevent inhaling the unwanted fragrances. The aisles of supermarkets are filled with soaps and shampoos that have their own distinct fragrances that were artificially added to them. For someone who showers, shampoos, shaves, and then uses hair gel and lotion—there are already five different fragrances that one is covered with.

The gustatory excess. Then there is the overstimulation of the taste buds. The food industry has figured out exactly what makes our mouths water, and what makes us consciously and unconsciously seek out certain foods. These "substances" have been refined, isolated, mass-produced and added to our foods for the sole purpose of whetting the appetite.

An example is the chemical MSG. Despite its well-known numerous side-effect, such as headaches and inability to concentrate due to excitotoxicity to the human nerve cells, they are present in nearly all canned soups and instant noodles. The use of these flavor-enhancing chemicals is more cunning than the old "restaurant trick" where the restaurateurs try to add maximum amounts of fat, salt and sugar to make the dishes taste better. The food manufacturing industry has succeeded in having teased out specific chemical components that will trigger appetite. Such artificially refined chemicals trigger appetite in people who honestly don't need any more calories. These chemicals are so common in the foods that we encounter on a daily basis that sometimes are impossible to avoid them altogether.

The five senses are heavily bombarded with stimulation from all sources. It is not that the use of five senses is inherently harmful. It is simply that the five senses are overtaxed to the point where the sixth sense is dwarfed.

The breakthrough insights are in the realm of the sixth sense

The five senses–visual, auditory, kinesthetic, olfactory and gustatory—are constantly kept busy and over-stimulated.

Revving the five senses in a constantly stimulated state comes at a heavy cost. One becomes disconnected from the sixth sense—the sense that is merely a "faint knocking" in comparison to the "loud" five senses.

The Boy And The Wristwatch

A little boy loses his wristwatch at home, and he is in a state of distress from the loss. The father discovers that the watch was lost in the living room, and comes up with an ingenious solution to solve the problem. The father turns off the TV and the fan, and everything else that makes noise. Then the father and the son both listen carefully for the ticking sound from the wristwatch. In that silence, they hear the faint ticking sound of the boy's wristwatch coming from the couch. The boy and the father find the wristwatch and celebrate their small victory.

The TV, the fan, and everything else stimulate the five senses. Trying to hear the inspiration is like trying to hear the faint wristwatch ticking. We need to quiet the five senses. Our true amazing potentials are expressed when our five senses calm down enough to allow us to reach beyond what see, hear, touch, smell and taste. The "volume" of an insight is so *sub-tle* that it requires us to quiet down the noise from the five senses in order for us to sense it.

Many live as if they had wisdom of their own.
Heraclitus

Being able to survive is praiseworthy, but being able to thrive is magnificent. It is because thriving can only come after mastering survival. Surviving has to do with meeting the basic needs—such as food, shelter and clothing. It is a form of existence, but nothing more. People who are in the survival mode tend to live a life of instinct.

Thriving, on the other hand, has to do with already having the basic needs of the physical body met. When such basic needs are met, one tends to live a life beyond the raw animal instincts, but rather a life of inspiration.

It is important to be in the state of thriving. It is during one's thriving times that there is the ample energy and inspiration to make things happen that would please the soul. The things that one creates during the thriving state become the worthy contributions to the world. In the state of thriving, one leaves a legacy behind.

Heraclitus is a presocratic Greek philosopher known for his statement; "No man ever steps into the same river twice." Heraclitus spoke of a spiritual quality called *Logos*, which is equivalent to the modern word, wisdom.

Heraclitus said that Logos, or wisdom *belongs to the common*. It is by its nature present everywhere. Logos allows a person to have the breakthrough insights necessary for one's transformation. Logos is open to people to tap into it.

According to Heraclitus, humanity has only a *minimum* amount of wisdom. Heraclitus says that the Logos is "all around us," but not "of us." The human body is not meant to be a source of wisdom, but rather an instrument of wisdom.

We can view the relationship between *humans* and *Logos* as that of a *radio* and the *broadcasted information* on the radio channels. The radio simply taps into the various radio stations already available to it. The radio is not the source of information. It merely channels the information. It can tune into the station that broadcasts the current traffic condition, the breaking news, the classical music, or an inspiring lecture. But one cannot confuse the receiver with the information, which the receiver channels.

I watched on a DVD of Jiddu Krishnamurti giving a seminar in 1985, a year before he passed away. He sat on a humble wooden chair upon an opera stage, and he would often become silent and raise his head to his side as if he is trying to hear something from the above. He would speak with many pauses, and spoke when he seemed *compelled* to say what he had just "heard." Could this be the secret to his deeply insightful revelations that he was known for?

I once heard Dr. Dietrich Klinghardt MD giving a presentation about the shape of human anatomical design. Did you know that our Atlas, the first neck bone, is shaped in the form of a parabolic antenna facing the sky above? Did you know that our feet standing shoulder-width apart also form a parabola facing the Earth? Perhaps these are simple coincidences, but to this author, these coincidences are the universe's reminder that humanity is a radio receiver ever so ready to channel the inspirations that are available all around us. Just as the radiowaves are not picked up on the radios that are not tuned into them, so is the wisdom of the universe, which cannot be picked up by those who are not tuned into it.

In our hectic daily lives, wisdom slips us by while we are consumed by the dramas of life. The stillness needed to hear the profound insights is impossible in a lifestyle dominated by the five-senses.

We are creative beings. We are evolving beings. Because of that, we need to have some moments of *stillness* between *movements* and *silence* between the *noises* of the five senses. It is in those precious moments of stillness and silence, do we access the vast wisdom of the universe, and gain precious life-transforming insights.

Sixth sense taps into the streaming of information that is beyond the detection of the five senses. It is in the realm of the sixth sense that one derives powerful insights and inspirations.

Actions turn an insight into a reality

An insight reveals what is clearly a possibility. Therefore, having the insight is having *half done*. The other half is to actively manifest it. For Michelangelo, seeing David in a flash of insight in a block of marble was only *half* the experience. Michelangelo had to work on the block of marble for three years to transform it into the 17-foot masterpiece sculpture of David[4].

Hear the beautiful voice of Tagore in his moving poem, *Waiting*.

I have spent my days
Stringing and unstringing my instrument;
While the song I came to sing
Remains unsung.
Rabindranath Tagore

Before we run out of time to do what we came to Earth to do, *sit*. Learn to *still* the mind, as calm as a calm lake that reflects the moon in one unbroken totality. Know that all is well in divine perfection. Let the highest levels of wisdom and inspiration *bathe* the psyche. Be connected to the Great Spirit—to hear the soft gentle voice that reminds you *why* your spirit decided to come to Earth. You want to be healthy—so that the diseases do not distract you from the path you came to tread.

The agony of incompletion is a burden to our minds. That is why we spend enormous amounts of time seeking closure for the past events in our lives. We all have come to Earth with a potential. We wish to sow our potential, and see it manifesting. We don't want to have the *unsung* songs still buried in our hearts when death comes for us.

As Tagore may agree, we don't want to keep busy for the sake of being busy, losing focus as to why we are "tuning" our instrument. When we are deaf to our own soul's calling, the beautiful song of life that we came to *sing* cannot be sung. The unique gifts and talents that we are to deliver to our world remain *undelivered.*

Time does not stop. Time seems cold and indifferent to people's needs or desires. Before life comes to an end, *sing* your heart's song. It is better to make mistakes than never having attempted. No one is skillful the first time. It takes practice to become skilled at anything. Malcolm Gladwell's best-selling book, *Outliers* explains that to be a master in anything, one simply needs to allocate 10,000 hours to practicing it. What a relief. All you need is to give it some time. Anyone can do it. You don't need to have the talent or genetics. It is the actions that turn your insights into a reality.

The top ten killers are heavily influenced by one's lifestyle

When life turns rotten, people blame their parents.
When life turns fantastic, people take the credit.
A Korean proverb

It is not the genetics why people become ill. Rather it is often the accumulation of years of unhealthy lifestyle habits. Let's look at the top ten causes of mortality on Table 1.

The top ten causes of death include heart disease, cancer, stroke, and diabetes, to name a few[5,6]. The surprising finding is that most of these diseases are neither genetic nor environmental, but rather considered *lifestyle diseases*. In other words, these top ten diseases—that likely will cause you and your loved ones the agonizing suffering—are a direct result of years of practicing unhealthy habits. These diseases are not a result of genetic disorder, malnutrition, pollution, or infection. In most cases, they are, and always have been, under *one's own* control. Thus, one's health is determined by one's actions. There is something very *liberating* about this fact. It's because this means that *patients* are in charge. When one is in charge, the individual can make changes to manifest the desired outcome.

Table 1. The top ten causes of death in U.S. 2006.[7]

Rank	Cause of death	% Total
1	Heart disease	26.0
2	Cancer	23.1
3	Stroke	5.7
4	Lung disease	5.1
5	Accidents[8]	5.0
6	Diabetes	3.0
7	Alzheimer's	3.0
8	Influenza and pneumonia	2.3
9	Kidney failure	1.9
10	Blood infection	1.4

Spend a majority of your time doing actions that are
Goal-achieving, and not tension-relieving.
Dr. Denis Waitley

A psychologist, and the best-selling author of *Psychology of Winning,* Dr. Denis Waitley, has said that successful people are the ones who distinguish themselves from others by spending a majority of their time doing actions that are *goal-achieving*, rather than *tension-relieving*.

So what is the key in creating and maintaining a healthy body? They have healthy habits.

Healthy people regularly exercise. Healthy people have hobbies. Healthy people walk daily. Healthy people floss their teeth. Healthy people eat breakfast and are significantly less likely to become obese or diabetes[9]. Healthy people eat foods that contain omega-3 essential fatty acids. Healthy people get enough sleep. Healthy people have meaningful social ties.

Dr. David Jenkins PhD and the author of *Building Better Health* reports that the benefits of social ties include the following: having an access to physical support (such as cooking and running errands) when you are ill, emotional support (sharing a burden, and therefore reducing it), and critical information (such that one becomes convinced to take positive steps towards successful life). *Healthy people, in other words, make a habit of doing things that unhealthy people simply don't do.*

Healthy people have built habits of doing actions that are productive and constructive towards health. An individual has the ability to overcome illnesses and manifest health and vitality by making *healthier choices.*

There is a race between healing and injury

If one has a cut on the finger, it will eventually heal. However, if one makes a cut into a piece of steak, it will not heal—no matter what treatments it receives. The body heals from injuries as long as one is alive.

The reason why the finger heals but not the steak is due to a *race* that goes on only during the time when one is still alive. It is a race between two powerful forces. One is the force of healing mechanism. The other is the force of injuries that accumulate in the body.

To illustrate this, picture a racetrack with two cars. The first car represents your *healing mechanism,* and the second car represents all the *injuries added to the body.*

The two cars have been racing since one's birth. When the two cars are at par, healing and injury are in a balance. When the car of injury is winning, the body breaks down because it cannot heal fast enough. When the car of healing is winning, one heals. Death is when the injury takes off too far, and healing cannot catch up to the rate of injuries. The race is on while one is alive—and the healing mechanism needs the support from the person to outpace the speed of injury.

The car of healing tends to outpace the car of injury—until about 25 years of age[10]. Then the car of injury begins to take off. The unhealthy lifestyle habits at one point had little health consequence. But after 25, unhealthy habits do cost dearly—in various symptoms such as headaches, lethargy and backpains just to name a few.

The solution to overcoming diseases and achieving health is simple. Support your healing while slowing down all injuries.

Joint injuries can be cured if treated early

Floss only the teeth that you want to keep, and forget the rest.
Zig Zigler

A big part of this author's personal passion is in treating *joint diseases*. These include back pain, hip joint pain, neck pain, elbow pain, shoulder injuries and ankle sprains. Typically, there are two areas that can cause problems in a joint—the *stabilizers* and the *cushions*.

The stabilizers are the *ligaments*. They keep the bones moving in a predetermined plane of motion. Picture how a typical door opens and closes. The *ligaments* act much like how *door hinges* "hold" the door onto the wall frame while allowing the door to move freely in a particular plane. If the door hinge is damaged, the door begins to creak and wobble as you try to open or close it. An injured ligament leads to the *wobbling* of the joint. Injured ligaments are painful because of the abundance of pain nerves in them. When a ligament is injured, the body will recruit the muscles around that ligament to "splint" the joint, thus to prevent further tearing of the ligaments. Without the splinting, the bones could eventually fall apart at the joint—just like the door falling off the wall frame because of the damaged hinge. To achieve this splinting, the body make the muscles go into spasm. A spasming muscle causes further problems, as the tendons of those contracted muscles tend to tear upon sudden movements, effectively spreading a ligament problem into a tendinosis problem. Since muscles use up a lot of energy trying to stabilize a joint, the affected person becomes quite fatigued over time.

The second thing that can go wrong in a joint is the *cushion* between the bones at the joint. This cushion is known as the *cartilage*. A cushion is necessary to prevent the painful *bone-to-bone* contact because the surface of the bone, known as the periosteum, is like a thin plastic wrap that is wrapped around the bone. This periosteum is highly loaded with nerve fibers that transmit pain signals when triggered. If you have ever had a broken bone, you know the pain the author is discussing. A bone should never weight-bear on another bone without cartilage to serve as a cushion between them.

This author often has patients referred to him for cartilage injuries to the knee. Unlike a *ligament* injury, a *cartilage* damage is much more difficult to heal. The condition suddenly deepens when we move from a ligament injury to cartilage injury; an analogy would be the floor of a fjord suddenly dropping into an abyss. When a joint has ligament problems that are not healed in time, it will eventually turn into cartilage damage. It is straightforward to resolve ligament tears through proper ligament realigning immediately followed by a procedure called *Prolotherapy*, and a few weeks of bracing. It often takes about five treatments, each a week apart, and the normal joint stability returns beautifully along with the disappearance of pain.[11] That window of opportunity can be lost if proper procedures are not performed in time.

When the ligaments are injured, the unstable joint begins to wobble excessively and the cartilage begins to *grind* whenever bone-to-bone friction occurs. When a joint has a ligament injury, even regular activities such as hiking and running can quickly grind up the cartilage, leading to a condition called osteoarthritis.

I see these cases all the time. What had been something very simple—a ligament has been partially torn—turns into an incurable condition—such as a cartilage tear over time.

There is the right time for everything. This very moment may be just the perfectly ripe time for your healing.

Health and fitness are two different things

Health and fitness are considered synonyms. However, there is a major difference between health and fitness. While health refers to the overall reliability of the body from breaking down, fitness refers to the overall performance potential of the individual. That is why one can be healthy, but not particularly fit. Conversely, one can be fit, but not exactly healthy. Let me explain with an analogy using a car.

If you are planning to choose a vehicle based on racetrack results, you may be confusing vehicle's *performance* with its *reliability*. For example Land Rover, Porsche, Alfa Romeo and Ferrari are all known to be super handling, highest performing vehicles. But they are not traditionally reliable vehicles as reported by Britain's insurance company, Warranty Direct[12].

When you are choosing a vehicle, you should look for its performance *and* reliability. The physical body also needs both—fitness and health.

One can be healthy, but not very fit. My maternal grandma was very healthy. She lived a healthy, disease-free life well into her 90's. But I wouldn't have asked her to run a marathon. She wasn't fit.

I knew a gentleman who can benchpress 315 pounds—a very strong man. But he was riddled with joint pains, headaches, lethargy, obesity and hypertension. He was an example of a man who was fit, but not healthy.

The ideal condition is to be both fit *and* healthy. A reasonable fitness is being able to lower heart rate by at least 30 beats per minutes after a 10-minutes intensive exercise such as stationary bicycling. To do this test, get on a stationary bicycle and pedal as hard as you can for 10 minutes. Measure your heart rate the moment you stop. This is simple if you have a heart rate monitor on your bicycle. Record the heart rate the moment you stop the 10-minute full out bicycling. Then exactly 1 minute after do the second reading. If your heart rate did not drop by *30 beats*, you are "out of shape." If the "recovery heart rate" is reduced by 30 beats or more, then you are considered "fit."

If you don't have an access to a heart rate monitor, you can get a reasonably good measurement by checking your pulse for 6 seconds at the same time you stop cycling, and multiply that number by ten. For example, let's say that as soon as you ended the 10-minute full out cycling, you checked your pulse on your neck, and you counted 19 beats over 6 seconds. 19 beats x 10 = 190 beats per minute. Therefore, your heart rate immediately after a 10-minuite full out cycling was 190 beats per minute. After exactly 1 minute, you counted 14 beats over 6 seconds, which means your recovery heart rate was 140 beats per minute. Since your drop in heart rate is 190 -140 = 50, your heart is considered to be in a good shape[13].

Do not do this test if you are suffering from a heart disease. You should check with your doctor first. On top of your recovery heart rate being 30 beats per minute less than during your very high intense exercise, there are three more things to check. All of the below, your doctor can find out for you. If you are an adult female, your ideal BMI is between 19-25.

BMI is *inaccurate* for people who are still growing, and men who are very muscular.

If you are an adult male, check for your body fat percentage, and if you are below 20% of body fat, you are in very good shape.

Your waist should be 50% or less of your height.

So that is fitness. But how do you measure health? Any studies that I have seen try to measure health in terms of fitness or longevity. However, one can be fit, but regularly misses school or work because of nagging headaches, allergies or colds. Or one may live a long life, but again frequented by numerous illnesses that are only controlled by dozens of powerful medications and frequent visits to the hospital emergency ward.

So how do you measure your health? For the time being, the only way is a subjective way. A healthy body *is* a reliable body that runs expectedly with very little maintenance—other than needing to provide it with the proper nutrients. A healthy body is a reliable body. Just like a reliable vehicle, a healthy body does not keep breaking down or require constant attention. When your body is relatively free of needing attention other than needing the occasional colds and flues, you can consider your body as healthy.

The forgotten ingredients for an extraordinary life

What did you do today that makes you wise, loving or courageous?
What did you do today that makes you wise, loving and courageous?

An extraordinary life involves the mastery in three ingredients of life. The three ingredients are wisdom, compassion and courage. Wisdom, compassion and courage make up the triune that an extraordinary life stands on. Having just one of these three "triune virtues" is considered incomplete for creating an extraordinary life. An extraordinary life requires all three at the same time.

A truly mature person demonstrates all three—wisdom, compassion and courage

In the African savanna, a wildebeest is born. This young offspring can walk within minutes. Under two hours it runs alongside head-to-head with the adult wildebeests to escape predators.

It is said that a human being becomes an adult upon reaching19 years of age. The government seems to believe this. At the age of 19, one is considered an adult and becomes legally responsible for one's actions.

But people mature at different rates. Some 15 year olds seem to have fully awakened into an adult, and he or she is already far on the great path living an extraordinary life. Then there are some 50 year olds who seem to have gotten lost along the way, and going through the *second* puberty. Clearly, biological age is not the sole criterion that distinguishes a grown-up from a child.

One of the *measuring sticks* that can differentiate an adult from a child is one's mastery over the triune virtues of wisdom, compassion and courage. Therefore, the ingredients for an extraordinary life also are the ingredients for a true adult. This is because an extraordinary life is only reserved for a true grown-up. Life provides ample opportunities for an individual to demonstrate and cultivate one's level of mastery over these triune virtues.

Wisdom—the first ingredient for an extraordinary life

Stay alert, stay alive.
Motto of the U.S. First Infantry Division in Vietnam

Wisdom is typically defined as one's ability to utilize knowledge. However, there is a precise definition for the word, *wisdom* that is used in this book. *Wisdom* is defined as *one's ability to protect oneself* from others. If one is not able to protect oneself from others, the person cannot be said to be wise.

In one's daily life, if the person encounters one hundred people, ninety-nine[14] of them are likely good or neutral, but there may be one person out of the hundred who is harboring a harmful mindset. Such a person is harmful to others. A *wise* person recognizes the harmful one from the crowd, and avoids interacting with this person. However, if there was no opportunity to avoid this harmful person, a wise person comes up with a clever way to escape the harm.

A clever fox outwits the tiger

One day the fox was walking through the forest, and suddenly ran into a very hungry tiger. The tiger said to the fox, "I'm sorry, but I haven't had anything to eat, so I will have to eat you. I hope you don't take it personally."

The fox, being clever and wise, decided not to let this day his last day on Earth. He used his sharp mind for his advantage.

He replied to the tiger, "I see. You obviously don't know me very well. Though I'm small, I assure you that I am the most ferocious animal in the jungle, and if I were not so generous in my heart, I could make you suffer the most horrendous death!"

This got the tiger's attention. The tiger was very hungry and tired, and the last thing it wanted was a lot of trouble for a meal. Still skeptical, the tiger replied, "Oh, really? I never heard that a little fox could do that. I am the tiger, and I am supposed to be the most ferocious!" The fox replied without a moment of hesitation, "That is why you are not the brightest. Let me prove it to you. Follow me, and just watch what happens when the forest animals see me."

Without a pause, the fox began walking ahead, and the tiger followed a few steps behind the fox. The tiger was fully alert, skulking, and looking around with its big bulging eyes for signs that may prove or disprove the fox's claim.

And, sure enough, the whole forest suddenly became chillingly silent. All the animals scurried away quickly or hid under the foliage holding their breaths as they saw the odd scene of the fox leading the tiger. Even the great elk and mighty bear took off in a hurry, not wanting to be spotted by the nasty tiger. No one wanted to risk any trouble with the tiger.

But seeing the reaction of the forest animals, the tiger thought it was the fox that they were all scared of. The tiger realized what grim trouble he had gotten himself into, and ran for his life to save himself from a certain horrendous death.

It is a story for children, but with a powerful lesson that can transform a child into an adult. Wisdom is needed to protect oneself from the predators. The world is a great place to live. The twenty-first century is perhaps the most prosperous years humanity has ever encountered, and we are all so lucky to be born in this tremendous period. However, it still has some dull beings that are destructive and predatory. You hear about them in the news for their heinous crimes, though they are perhaps somewhat over-represented in the media.

"First cultivate your wisdom," said the sages. Protect yourself from harm, so that you can lead a life of your choice.

Once you have wisdom, you move onto developing compassion.

Compassion—the second ingredient for an extraordinary life

With spiritual ascension, a common passion
Matures into an uncommon compassion.

The second virtue of a mature being is compassion. Compassion and passion are differentiated in terms of their level of maturity. Passion is the mindset of a *beginner*. Passion is necessary for one to get started and get moving. It is a powerful motivator, but it is still an immature emotion that is in need of growing into its mature form—compassion.

So how do the ancient sages define compassion?

Compassion is your ability to protect your loved ones from *you*!

Being blinded by passion, one cannot see the viewpoints of others. The mind becomes rigid and polarized. Stress level rises. Adrenaline floods the veins. Pupils dilate. Breathing becomes heavy. Heart pounds. Muscles shake. Strain in the psyche disables the reasoning mind. This is when one can cause the most harm to others. For example, have you ever heard of a "compassionate terrorist?" There is no such a thing. Terrorists are passionate people who cannot see from any other person's perspective outside of their own. Blinded by passion, they cross over a line that they should not have crossed. Examine the passionate quote from Hammurabi. Compare that with the compassionate response of Gandhi.

An eye for an eye.
The Codes of Hammurabi of 1780 BC, by Hammurabi the King of Babylonia.

An eye for an eye makes the world go blind.
Gandhi (1869-1948), the peaceful liberator of India.

Metaphorically speaking, you are 99 percent of the time compassionate or neutral, but 1 percent of the time you are in a weakened state. You lose your inner strength and become completely (and with much reduced IQ) passionate. We've all been there, and probably got our "T-shirts" too, to show that we've been there and done that.

We end up becoming small and petty. We are filled with jealousy, fear and disappointment, and we lash out.

But to whom?

Almost always to the ones those are dear to us. These are the people whom you should never lash out to! These are your loved ones—your loving spouse, your precious children, and the irreplaceable supporters and well-wishers in your life. When people are intimate, they have the "access key" to their loved one's inner vulnerable core. What you say can hurt or heal with impact thousands of times more—compared to what any strangers can. The family and friends are the anchors and cheerleaders of one's life!

And it's sad, but typically the family and friends are exactly the ones who are also the ones we tend to lash out to in our unbridled passion. In the moment of passion, the reason is clouded, and we lose our center.

Compassion is your ability to put up a *protective shield* around your loved ones. You'd put this protective shield on them in order to protect them from *you*! It is a shield to protect your loved ones from your inability to control your own raw, passionate outbursts. You know what it is like when you have been a victim of such a raw outburst from your loved ones. It is always regretful to hurt our loved ones, and regretful to have been a victim of such harsh, toxic energy.

A word on passion. Generally speaking, having passion is a good thing. But an *unbridled* passion is dangerous—like riding in a powerful vehicle that has no steering system. Remember, compassion is made up of two words, *com* and *passion.* When we are compassionate, we *study* the passion of everyone involved. Once we take the "pulse" of the group, we become aware of their pains and pleasures, and begin to understand their needs. This is the state where compassion can arise.

Courage—the third ingredient of an extraordinary life

The knowledge of HOW does not come before the ACTION, but only after.
Bob Proctor

You can always tell when someone lacks courage. He has a habit of making "How do I do it?" types of remarks. Courage is our ability to overcome our fears and do something that we believe to be the right thing to do.

At the most crucial moment to commit oneself into action, an individual who lacks courage says, "I don't know *how* to do this." Not everything in life is like the new IKEA furniture that comes with the instruction manual. There are many things in life that require you to *do* it first, before you find out the *how*. You don't have to pioneer everything, but if you are an individual seeking growth, you would inevitably run into an unexplored territory. It is at these times, you would have to exercise the courage that you have cultivated.

Sir Edmund Hillary is a perfect example of someone who mastered this virtue of courage.

Sir Edmund Hillary's victory

Total understanding =
Theoretical understanding + experiential understanding.

Some people go to school and gain theoretical knowledge.

Then they go out into the workforce and gain experiential knowledge. Others go and gain experimental knowledge. Then after they have done it, they come up with a theory. Either way, the total and complete understanding requires the person to walk the same path twice—once in mind and the second time in body.

Benefiting from those who have come before, most fields of knowledge already have become well established with well-organized theories that provide the "map' for those new initiates to navigate more easily and safely. Those new initiates are riding on the coattail of those who have trail blazed the field before them. One such pioneer is Sir Edmund Hillary.

When Edmund Hillary climbed Mount Everest, he didn't know *how* to climb this tallest mountain in the world. There existed no record of anyone who had succeeded it before him and left behind a map to help climb this mountain. Previous to Hillary, ambitious mountaineers either have failed or died trying. It was said at the time that the very air one breathes at the peak of Mount Everest could kill the person because of the low concentration of oxygen! So what made Hillary so special that he thought he could climb to the top of the world? After all, he was just a beekeeper from New Zealand!

But Edmund Hillary conquered it with his Nepali guide, Tenzing Norgay, and stood on top of the world on May 29, 1953! After having successfully conquered what had been thought impossible, he probably told himself, "Now I know *how* to climb Mount Everest."

That is right. You can understand mountain climbing in theory first and then in action later, or you can understand it experientially first by action and then in theory after.

People often harbor the mistaken concept that they must know *how* to do something before they actually do anything. They want to be led by their hand through every new thing in their lives. But this is certainly not the path of a courageous soul. There are occasions that life calls out to a person for an adventure. Everyone is capable of trailblazing a new territory and creating the map for others behind, and add to the collective human knowledge.

A mature person masters all three virtues

A person of wisdom, compassion, and courage is well centered. However, the three virtues are like the legs of a tripod, which have to stay together as a unit and work in harmony. When separated, they become unbalanced, unstable and tip over.

Imagine a person who is quite wise, so he is able to protect himself, but lacks compassion for others. This fits a profile of a heartless psychopathic *gang leader*. With the power of his wisdom, he manipulates others in order to secure power for his own sake. Wisdom on its own is *monstrosity*.

Then imagine a person who lacks wisdom, but is full of compassion. This is a profile of a *fool*. He will be taken advantage by everyone who is desperate enough to do so, and therefore, leads a life of constantly being used and abused.

Or imagine a person who has both wisdom and compassion, but lacks courage for action. He would be a person who has all the positive and brilliant solutions to the world's problems, but is never able to solve any of them because he is paralyzed by fear. You have met this type. He talks a good talk, but fails to move into a meaningful action. If you ask him what he has done, he can only tell you of his magnificent plans, but that is all he can offer to the world. The chance of carrying out the plans may long have passed him by.

An enlightened person is someone who has gone back to become a child, *tzu*

"Truly I tell you, anyone who will not receive the kingdom of God like a little child will never enter it."
Mark 10:16

Life is filled with irony. A person who has demonstrated wisdom, compassion and courage is a true grown-up. However, when such grown-up fully masters the triune virtues, he becomes *childlike*.

In the Western tradition, Jesus said that *to enter the kingdom of God, one needs the attributes of a little child.* Coincidentally, in the Eastern tradition a person who has reached the enlightenment is given the title "*child*." In the Classical Chinese, word for "child" is "*tzu*." So there is *Kongtzu* (Confucius), *Laotzu*, *Motzu* (Mozi) and *Mengtzu* (Mencius)—indicating that they all have reached their enlightenment. A deeper analysis of the word, "tzu" reveals that it is a compound word made up of two separate words. They are the word "one" and the word "done."

子 = 一 + 了

子 *is pronounced "tzu"; a Chinese character for "child."*

一 *is pronounced "yi"; a Chinese character for "one."*

了 *is pronounced "liao"; a Chinese character for "done."*

The word "*tzu*" then literally is a title given to an individual who has discovered the "one thing" that matters most to the person, pursued it, and has *done it*. In the Eastern tradition, it is considered that one has reached the enlightenment when one has done that one thing that matters the most. By virtue of having reached enlightenment, the person attains the higher state of vibration that is commonly associated ironically—with a child. Life seems *circular* in nature.

From the "blank innocence" to "mature innocence"

A human child starts out its life marked by innocence. It is what children are known for. However, a child is innocent by default. A child does not know any other way, but to be innocence. Then soon, a child begins to show a strong affinity to one of the three virtues. One child, for example, is naturally wise—it can protect itself. It can talk its way out of any difficult situation. Another child is naturally compassionate—it can protect its loved ones. It shows a great deal of care and love towards others. Yet another child is naturally courageous—it constantly challenges the limits of its fears. It is able to do things that it does not know how.

Any child starts out life with strength in one of the three triune virtues. However, until the child develops proficiency in the other two of the triune virtues, the child is not considered a grown-up. A grown-up is autonomous by definition, and a child who lacks even one of triune virtues is either a danger to itself or others.

Consider a child who is naturally wise, but lacks compassion. It is merely a cold manipulator. Consider another child is naturally compassionate, but lacks wisdom. It is merely a fool who gets abused constantly. Consider a third child who is naturally courageous, but has neither wisdom nor compassion. It is merely a brute who gets manipulated into doing harmful things to self and others.

When an individual demonstrates all three virtues, he is considered from that point on, a grown-up. The grown-up at one point begins to yearn for innocence, and one day takes the leap and reaches innocence for the second time. This second innocence is known as the *mature* innocence. This individual then has reached the state that meets the criterion to the title of *tzu*—which is another title for a *saint*.

An act of compassion and courage in a third grader

Jua was in Grade 3, and she had to do a weather report presentation in class—supposed to announce the weather like a professional TV weather forecaster. The ones who were presenting had to go up to the front of the class and include in the presentation two things—the weather condition and temperature—in order to get an A grade.

The first kid went up, and forgot to mention the weather condition. The second kid got up, and forgot to mention the temperature. The third kid got up to present only to forget both, and so on. Then Jua got up and forgot the temperature. Later on, Jua's mom asked her why she didn't do it right even though she did her homework and practiced so well at home. Jua replied that she didn't want to make her friends feel stupid by her getting it perfect.

Jua demonstrated compassion for her classmates who failed and lost face. She also showed courage to do what she thought was the right thing to do. She stood up and *intention-*

ally made the mistake and looked foolish. She *does* lack the development of wisdom, but she is only in third grade. She will, no doubt master wisdom in no time.

Such marvelous level of awareness from a mere third grader! She has demonstrated a rare level of proficiency in compassion *and* courage.

According to Buddhism, humans have infinite potential to *know* anything, to *do* anything, to *have* anything.

In fact, a Buddhist would say that one already *knows* everything. The reason why one cannot yet recall everything is because of the "clouds" that cover one's true nature of all potentiality.

Socrates says of education that people already have the infinite knowledge, which is innate to them, and an outstanding teacher is someone who helps the student to realize that the student already *knows* everything.

"Educo" means to *lead out*—to lead out the knowledge inherent within the student. In fact, *education* must be differentiated from mere *training*. While education focuses on leading out the knowledge that the student already has, training is *imposing* a specific piece of knowledge on the student. When a school system is focused simply on imposing information and data on the students, it is merely engaged in training, not education.

Socrates argued that if a person didn't already knew something, he would not recognize it even if it stood in front of him. He continued that if he saw his old friend in a market place, he would recognize the friend only because he already *knew* the friend. If he didn't know the friend, there would no recognition.

Therefore, if one recognizes the three virtues, it is because one already has it within himself. All one needs to do is to draw out these secret ingredients of an extraordinary life. Then one needs to practice these triune virtues to the level of mastery. Practicing transforms what is awkward into something graceful.

Humans are capable of continued growth

Growth involves entering into *terra incognita*—the land of the unknown. The new territory one steps into has no map. Therefore, one is bound to make mistakes.

Mistakes and failures are not signs of a descent—but rather signs of an *ascent*. Look at the best baseball players in the Major League. If they hit three out of ten, they are doing extremely well. If they are consistently able to hit four times out of ten, they will be considered one of the best in baseball history. One can fail six times out of ten and he is considered the greatest!

People have the most powerful *tool* already—time. Regardless of one's wealth, health, gender or socio-economic status, everyone gets the equal amount of time—*the twenty-four hours in a day*. Being smarter or wealthier does not provide one with more hours in a day.

This is a relief.

In fact, all the necessary conditions that the highly functioning person has, the least functioning person has too. They are playing on the same level fields with neither having more nor less of the essentials. These include time, space, air and gravity. The highly functioning individuals simply make a more effective use out of these basic, essential resources.[15]

A life truly worth living is worth recording

Life surprises us with flashes of insight. As quickly as they came, they quickly disappear into oblivion. A handheld journal can record these insights that later can be reorganized into a meaningful perception of the world that one lives in.

It is often said that humans are *blessed* because they *forget*—so that they can forget their painful memories. That may perhaps be the case. If that logic is sound, humans must also be *cursed* because they forget their happy memories. Aside from being a blessing or a curse, one is faced with a fact that the human memory is imperfect. It is to one's advantage to remember what he finds valuable, and disregards those that he finds worthless.

The key to remembering is through recording and reciting. There is a simple law to overcoming bad memory. The law is this: Repetition Creates Memory. To remember the valuable insights in life, one simply needs to write down what one wishes to remember, and then recite repeatedly until it gets recorded in the permanent memory bank.

Record those rare thought gems *permanently* by writing them down in a designated hardbound journal book that can be carried around. A life worth living is worth recording.

To increase the mind power, one has to *decrease* the number of thoughts

The mind is a tool that can bring diffuse thoughts into a focus. Everyone has played with a magnifying glass as a child. Everyone would have realized that there are two things that must be done to obtain power from the magnifying glass. Power is realized when (1) the magnifying glass is brought into a *focus*, and (2) it is to *be still* at one spot and not moving it around.

The mind obtains power the same way. To obtain power from the mind, the mind requires (1) focused attention, and (2) being still and remaining at one spot. The thoughts are the movements of the mind. Once the mind is in focus, the mind needs to maintain its stillness and be focused on one spot.

People have many thoughts that go through the mind in a given day. There are often too many thoughts swimming around in one's mind, but worse yet, many of those thoughts are not even self-initiated. These thoughts neither have a clear purpose for the thinker, nor do they resolve any problems. They are just random, low-grade thoughts lacking power to inspire the thinker into action. They are not much useful, other than perhaps to provide feedback to the thinker that he lacks a clear focus in life. However, the mind is a powerful tool, but seriously under-utilized.

Imagine that a powerful deity appears one day, and says that from now on you are cursed to have only one thought for the rest of your life and you have five minutes to make your choice, what would be this *one thought* that you would choose? Would you choose a thought of anger, jealousy, fear, disappointment, or depression? Or would you rather choose a thought of peace, harmony, happiness, courage, wisdom or compassion?

A laser (Light Amplification by Stimulated Emission of Radiation) is light that has been focused and is therefore coherent and *self-converging*. It means that their photons align themselves into one sharp focused stream. This focused energy of normal visible light can cut through one the hardest known substances on Earth, such as diamonds and steel.

When the mind is focused, it acts like the laser beam. It accomplishes what is normally considered impossible. The laser-focused mind begins manifesting insights into reality. Mental discipline is an act of controlling the types of thoughts that one has.

To achieve health, keep in mind the thoughts of health. I have known people who claim to be "health conscious" but often fill their conversations with illnesses. Such a focused mind zoomed on illnesses is a mind that is leading the person to illnesses—not health. To achieve health, keep the mind on the various states of health—soaring energy, lean body, elastic skin, powerful muscle, flexible body, and slow and steady resting heart rate.

Helping children develop their three virtues

I often hear of table conversations that go like this:
Dad: How did your school go?
Son: All right I guess.
Dad: Anything happened?
Son: Well, nothing really.

Children often believe that the things that are worth telling adults should be "adult-worthy" things—factual and significant. I think it's because we ask them to do this as part of helping them develop a clear communication skill. But the message can be mistaken, as "adults don't want to hear the little things that happen to kids."

But when we trip over something, it is rarely a mountain that we trip over. It is usually a little rock or root sticking out of the ground that we have over-looked. When a relationship isn't going well, it isn't because of the big events, but rather the little things. A relationship is not built on the big events, but on those relatively little things in our lives. It's because the *small talks* reveal much about the speaker's mindset, and the direction that the speaker is looking.

What elevates our spirit is the level of the question that we have in our minds. Until a child can ask highly inspiring questions on their own, the parents can guide them to raise their level of awareness. Certainly, a conversation can be focused around the basic virtues of wisdom, compassion and courage. Here is an example.

Dad: What did you do that was courageous today? [This guides a child in a specific direction.]
Son: Oh, at lunchtime, I saw a kid getting bullied, and I helped him.
Dad: How did you manage that without getting injured yourself? [This is a question checking the level of his development in wisdom.]
Son: There were three of them, all mean-looking, and I didn't have anyone else to help me. The poor kid looked terrified, and I couldn't just pass by. So I thought about what I could do. I ran back into the school, and grabbed the first teacher I found, and told him what was going on. The teacher came out and took the bullies to the office.
Dad: That was quick thinking. So why did you decide to help the kid? [A question checking his development in compassion.]
Son: I know how scary it felt to be singled out like that. I didn't want that to happen to anyone.

In the 21st Century, perhaps the most dangerous place is the dining table. It has become a place where excess calories are consumed. The habitually excessive caloric consumption has led to the level of public health nightmare where over 30% of the population is obese. Obesity is a direct contributor to hypertension, high cholesterol and diabetes—and in turn open up a whole slew of diseases such as immune deficiency, kidney failures, blindness, heart attack, stroke, Alzheimer's and cancer.

May your dining table be transformed into a place of where you can nourish the body of every member of your family, but also their *mind.*

Unresolving stress is the health enemy number one

I gain much insight into the lifestyle of my patients when I see their cortisol panel. Cortisol is produced from the adrenal gland. It is a stress hormone, which reaches its highest level in the blood stream around 6 am, and steadily lowers each hour to its absolute lowest around 3 am the next morning. Then it begins increasing in amount again to its highest at 6 am.

Cortisol has two main functions. First it causes the liver to release the stored glucose into the blood stream. Therefore cortisol increases the blood glucose level. It is a little known fact, but the blood glucose is reserved only for the brain, and no other organ. The heart is not allowed to use glucose for energy. Neither is the liver allowed to use sugar. In fact, only the brain is allowed to burn glucose for energy[16]. Cortisol has a 24-hour rhythm, and it appears to strongly influence the sleep cycle. Cortisol level is the highest at 6 am, and in response to cortisol rise, the glucose level rises in the blood stream. The increase in blood glucose level provides more glucose for the brain. Thus, it provides enough energy for the brain to awaken from sleep.

Cortisol panel is done with saliva samples collected at 4 different times in one 24-hour period—at 6 am, 12 noon, 4 pm, 8 pm. The collection is done by collecting watery portion of saliva relatively free of mucus and foam. Mucus comes from the digestive system and lacks hormones. Foam has very little amount of actual saliva. The mouth should be free of any food. Therefore, the mouth should be rinsed only with clean water without brushing (to avoid bleeding). You should spit out as much water as possible, and wait 15 minutes before collecting about 5 ml. The sample should be frozen immediately.

Individuals who tend to wake up in the middle of the night should take one more collection when this occurs. For those who tend to wake up in the middle of the night, often it is a sudden rise in cortisol that causes blood glucose level to rise, and awaken the person.

The 4-point cortisol test can reveal important data about the level of stress the person has been under. Actually, it is more the level of the person's *perception* of stress, rather than stress itself. It is because the physiological reaction to stress depends on the individual *perception* of stress, rather than stress itself. To clarify this, let's take an example of encountering a dog. Person X sees a dog and enters into a state of *delight*. Person Y sees the same dog and enters into a state of *fright*. The actual stressor, in this case a mutt, plays some role, but the physiological reaction stems from one's perception.

Many patients who come in complaining of lack of energy have significantly reduced levels of cortisol production. Restoring the adrenal glands is slow and may take five years or more. Adrenal glands are a collection of nerve cells. Nerve cells recover relatively slower than other tissue types, such as intestinal cells or skin cells. Therefore, the key is in preventing the adrenal glands from going into the "burnout" stage.

Everything is made twice: once in mind, and then in form

A Zen student asked the Zen master, "Master, when is the best time to start?" *The master replied, "When you are finished, of course."*

This type of conversations is known as the *kong-an* or *koan* in Zen Buddhism. The meanings of koans are not easily understood by rational thinking, but should be deciphered through a direct experience or intuition.

What does it mean to *start* when you are *finished*? The rational mind may argue why you'd even need to start when you already are finished.

The meaning contained in the above koan becomes profound when you stop thinking, and actually start experiencing it. Let's explore this further.

In order to *start* building a solid house, first you need to be already have built the house *inside* your mind. In your mind, you would have already done your blueprint of how many bedrooms, bathrooms, the number of stories, and many others before you actually start digging.

Before one lifts a cutting saw, one should already have decided where to apply that saw on wood, or chaos ensues.

Buddhists say that there is a time for meditation and time for action. Action should only start when the meditation is complete. Thus, in order to create a masterpiece, there is *a time for meditation* and *a time for action*.

So when is the best time to start anything?

It is a marvel to see how high-rises get built. At one moment, you see nothing but a concept in someone's mind. Then, a blueprint. Then the permits. Then the bustling of construction workers on site. Then before you knew it, it is there! A high-rise where an empty space used to be. Now there occupies a solid structure that if you walked into it, you would bump your head.

And what started out as a mere thought in someone's head is now a concrete reality. What existed merely in the form of thoughts has become a physical fact.

Everything great is done twice: once in the mind, and then later in physical action. Health, also, cannot be left to chance. You first envision it, and then make it come true.

We are One

Be humble that you are made up of the earth.
Be noble that you are made up of the stardust.

Give yourself a healthy self-worth. Self-esteem is made up of self-worth and self-confidence. Self-worth is an estimation how good one is without needing a proof; while self-confidence depends on your achievements and successes. With low self-worth, you may not have enough self-esteem to move on, discover, grow and master the unchartered territories of life.

I heard Dr. Deepak Chopra speaking sometime ago. He said that you are important because you are the *center* of the universe. You are the core around which the world revolves—just like what your mother made you believe when you were a child. Without you, your world is not complete.

Imagine yourself standing at the top of the world—Mount Everest—and visualize holding in your hands an immensely powerful laser gun that can shoot out a laser beam that can pierce through anything. In this scenario, activate this laser beam, and let it shine straight in front of you. How far will the laser beam go? Astronomers will tell you that it will peter out before reaching the end of the universe. But if it could, it would travel forever—towards *infinity*.

What if you send the laser beam to the exact opposite direction? Again, infinity.

How about to the top? How about to the bottom? If it could

penetrate through everything, in all directions, the laser beam will continue traveling forever. Because infinity extends from you in all directions in equal distance, mathematically, *you are the center of the universe*.

You are the center of the universe. That gives you one extra reason to be important! You can carry yourself with a sense of *dignity* and treat yourself with utmost royal *respect*.

But how about your best friend, let's say Steve, sitting at home studying his Quantum Physics at this very moment? Surely, infinity extends from him in all directions as well. So he is the center of the universe, too.

How about your cat, Fluffy, and your dog, Pepper? Aren't they also the rightful centers of their own universes? Treat them with the highest respect. In fact, let's treat everyone and everything with respect and awe. They are all the centers of the universe. If everyone is the center of the universe, that makes us all ONE.

In Hinduism, people greet each other with the word *namaste*. Namaste is literally translated as "*I bow to you.*" Of course, this "you" isn't your physical body nor your ego. This "you" is your highest self, your God-self. When you say namaste, you are really saying, "I see your God-self. You see my God-self. Let's resonate at that highest level." So here I go. Namaste!

Ultimately, our problem will be a problem of time—the lack of it

Dr. Joseph Campbell is the best-selling author of *The Hero's Journey*, *Hero with a Thousand Faces*, and *Power of Myth*. He had dedicated much of his life to studying Hinduism. It is a rich culture that parallels the sophistication of the Greek Mythology.

Hinduism has thousands of deities. So a question often rises. Of all these deities, who is the most powerful? In the Greek Mythology, the answer is clear. It is clearly Zeus. However, it isn't so clear in Hinduism.

Some believe the most powerful deity is *Brahma*, the creator god. Some claim that it is *Vishnu*, the preserver god. Still others say it is *Shiva*, the destroyer god.

The most powerful Hindu deity, in my opinion, must be *Kali*, the goddess of time. When she declares that *time is up*, even the great Brahma, Vishnu and Shiva have to pack up their bags and disappear into thin air.

The unstoppable and irreversible *passing of time* is one thing that we can all be certain of. Time does not stop, and we are always inching towards an end. An end to an illness. An end to a suffering!

To best make use this precious commodity, one must utilize the concept of timing. "Timing is everything," some say. Is there a difference between getting to the airplane 15 minutes too early versus 15 minutes too late?

Of course.

How about planting seeds a month too late in the season? You can have done everything right, but if you missed out on the timing, all your effort is lost, and ultimately there will be *no payoff*.

Diseases have the same pattern. If one hesitates a little too long, an otherwise *curable* condition degenerates into an *incurable* disease. It is especially heart-breaking if we discover that we are just a little too late.

Early type II diabetes, for example, is a simple problem that can be *cured* through a healthy diet, exercise and fat loss. In most cases, diabetes can be prevented altogether by eating whole foods, exercising regularly, and keeping your body at an ideal weight.

Once diabetes becomes full-blown, reversing it takes significantly more time and energy, but still may be curable.

However, if proper treatment is further delayed and crosses beyond the zone of healing, the diabetic patient can experience some permanent tissue changes. These changes result in the diabetic patient becoming blind or deaf, or they might need to have their feet amputated. Neuropathic pains down the legs, kidney failures, delirium and dementia can set in as well. These tissue changes signal that *the line* that separates a "curable" condition and "incurable" has been crossed. Treatments that would have worked previously will longer be effective.

Respect timing—so that recovering health is not too late. In reality, health is under the individual control. The solution to all diseases often is quite simple. Just by losing some fat, you can lower your blood pressure, cure diabetes, prevent heart disease, and avoid stroke.

As mentioned in previously in this book, Malcolm Gladwell, in his best-selling book, *The Outliers*, discusses Dr. Anders Ericsson's work (1990) that one can become an expert in anything if one *practices deliberately* for 10,000 hours. This equates to 20 hours of deliberate practice per week, for 50 weeks of the year for 10 years (20 x 50 x 10 = 10,000 hours). Dr. Ericsson's research brought out the importance of direct experience in acquiring mastery in a field as opposed to some innate ability that one is born with.

This concept of practicing 10,000 hours is both liberating and daunting at the same time. It is liberating if both Ericsson and Gladwell are correct because it means a person can master anything he chooses.

It is also daunting because if mastery takes 10,000 hours, which would roughly take 10 years, one must choose carefully. In order to devote 10 years per field, there isn't enough time to master perhaps more than a dozen fields in one's lifetime if we look at the human lifespan as 120 years, even if we maximized all those years and practiced your craft every single year without taking a break from them.

That is why we must meditate. Having a still mind can provide us with enough clarity to decide on the things that are worth spending our time while we are on Earth.

Existentialism

Existential philosophers believe in three things. These are:

1. We are thrown into this world, and we don't know why we are here.
2. We have the freedom to do whatever we desire.
3. Every action has a consequence that we must bear.

Everything meaningful is created twice. Once as a mental construct. The second as a reality. Reality is a concrete fact that can be verified by others. The grander the creation, the greater investment of time, energy and money that tend to be required.

Existential philosophers teach us that whether we like it or not, we own the consequences of our actions. Therefore, it is prudent to spend some time for meditation, and then spend time for action.

Of all the things you learn to master in this world, I suggest spending some time dedicated to learning the art of self-healing—starting, perhaps, with this book. Unless you'd like to gain enough knowledge and experience to treat others, a short-term dedication on the subject of *healing* for one year may suffice.

Consider the lilies of the field, how they grow;
They neither toil nor spin,
Yet I tell you, even Solomon in all his glory
Was not arrayed like one of these.
(Jesus, the Sermon on the Mount; Matthew 6:28–29)

You already have the most important things

You already have the most important things that no amount of money, energy or time could ever buy. Jesus was reassuring the crowd that the Universe has already taken care of humanity's basic needs for survival. The most important things for life are already provided. The air, water, and sunshine to grow crops are precious necessities and are already provided. Consider the riddle below.

The most expensive are the cheapest,
And the cheapest most expensive.

What is the thing that you own that had cost you the most?

According to 2008 Statistics, 30 percent of Canadians spent over their affordability threshold (determined by their household income) on acquiring their house between 2002 and 2004.[17,18] Spending over this threshold on a shelter is living beyond one's means.[19] This means that 30% of Canadians are going through mental strain just to pay for the mortgages. We, Canadians really seem to value our homes... If you'd ask a typical Canadian what is the most expensive thing that they possess, it would be reasonable to hear "home."

But if a house is burned down, you can still get another one—often a newer and perhaps even a better one. Usually your insurance will kick in, or you can apply your knowledge to get yourself one that is superior to the previous house.

In twenty-first century North America, with a little bit of self-discipline, you can earn significantly more than you spend. You can begin amassing material abundance. Of course, material abundance is just a collateral benefit that proves your strategies are working.

Jim Rohn, the author of *7 Strategies for Wealth & Happiness*, *My Philosophy for Successful Living*, and *Five Major Pieces to the Life Puzzle*, once said that everyone should focus on becoming a millionaire at least once. But *not* for the money. He says that you can give away the money. Rohn says that you should become a millionaire at least once for what the process *makes of you*. It takes a certain mental posture and self-control to achieve such an accomplishment. These include a powerful vision, clear goal setting, discipline and efforts carried out in an organized way.

With a crystal-clear vision to set your course towards your destination, and an intense focus to deal with immediate tasks on hand, you can conquer each step toward your predetermined goal. When you reach the goal, you'd have *become* a different person!

All the worldly rewards are just a bonus, like a good letter grade to prove to yourself that you understand your subject material. The world can take away from you everything you have gathered, but it can't take away the *person* that you have become.

The things that you paid the most for are relatively "cheap" in comparison to the things that have come to you *for free*.

You didn't pay for the air. Yet without it, you will die in five minutes.

Gravity: without it, you would float away into space.

Your family: your mother and father, your loved ones—none of them can be replaced with money or effort.

But once these are gone, no money in the world, or the efforts you put out, can ever bring them back to you.

The most important things in life that you need—air, sunshine, gravity, your physical body, your ability to heal yourself—*are given free of charge*. When it comes to the most important things in life, you are on equal footing with the most successful. Jesus, in the Bible, says to *consider the lilies, how they grow. They neither toil nor spin. But they are full of grace and grandeur!* You already have everything you need to succeed in life!

One of the "free," but most precious things of all is your *ability to heal yourself.* It is known in naturopathic medicine as *Vis Medicatrix Naturae*. It is translated as "The Healing Power of Nature." Your body has the ability to heal itself. This is the most powerful ally you can have to help you reach your health destination. Without this help, health would be impossible. You have this innate ability to heal available to you free of charge, 24 hours a day, 365 days a year!

The body heals itself. It is all *autonomic*. Autonomic is different from *automatic*. With automatic you still have to consciously be in control, while autonomic requires no conscious effort. For example, when you have a cut on your finger, it just heals without your conscious effort. The fact remains that the body is able to heal itself.

To assist healing, you need to give the body what it needs to heal, and get out of its way.

Your body runs on specific fuels and repairs itself with specific building blocks. The fuels are the carbohydrates and fats; and the building blocks are what we call *nutrients*—such as amino acids, essential fatty acids, minerals, vitamins, carbohydrates, water and oxygen. Give these to your body and let the body take care of the rest for you. The best thing that you can do is to remove the strains on the body while it tries to do its job.

When your body is seeking fresh fruits and vegetables, don't give it coffee and donuts and ask why the body is so slow in healing. The body is always trying to heal. When the body is suffering from an infection, and you ingest foods that are low in nutrients and sometimes downright toxic, your body may not *complete* its healing process.

Your body tries to heal by default, but when you keep interfering with it, you are not sending a crystal-clear message to your body. "Handsome is what handsome does." You do what is consistent with healing, and you will heal your illnesses and regain health.

You have a sophisticated healing system

You might already have realized how your body is truly an amazing machine. Each time I carefully examine it, I notice that the body makes the finest computers look like rusty nails in comparison. No matter how sophisticated, these man-made machines may never catch up to the human body in one crucial aspect—its ability to heal itself.

Your body's sophisticated *healing system* attempts to maintain itself in optimum health. Of course, you may wonder why, then, people are suffering from diseases when the body has such an incredible healing system.

In a majority of cases, your body's ability to heal has much to do with *your* behavior. The result of what you do can slow down or speed up your healing process.

Is your body stupid or do we simply not understand it? My good friend, a psychiatrist, Dr. Derek Neale once told me about a mildly retarded patient who felt unfairly treated by his family, saying, "Everyone keeps telling me that they don't *understand* me because I am so stupid. But, if they don't *understand* something, aren't they the stupid ones?"

His IQ test may have shown a lack in certain areas of intelligence, but this statement can only come from a highly thoughtful individual.

The same goes for the body's innate intelligence. It is superbly capable of maintaining life and healing. But it isn't explored in what is considered the "scientific" medicine. Just because we don't understand the mysteries of the body does not make the body a stupid piece of machinery.

A wise gardener asks you this question:

If the crops are failing to thrive in the garden, should you blame those crops?

Of course not.

A skilful gardener would choose to examine whether the conditions are optimum for the plants to thrive. However, the plants already have the ability to thrive. The problem nearly always is in the condition. There is something in the current condition that prevents the crops from thriving. He would ask whether there is too little or too much sunshine, too little or too much water. A wise gardener would not blame the plants for their failure to thrive.

The human folly is that we often lose faith too quickly; we walk into a cloud of uncertainty and become grabbed by discomfort and act in frustration. In fact, the same blaming attitude is sometimes seen in people treating their children, or their spouses.

A wise person must refrain from pointing fingers at living things. No living things should be subject to blaming or shaming.

Dr. Timothy Brown ND once said of his philosophy of "No blame; No shame." When something frustrates us, it is human nature to blame someone as the cause of the problem. Whe[illegible] this tactic doesn't work, the blaming person flips the ar[illegible] around and points the negative energy towards himse[illegible] pointing of negative energy is called shame. No living thing should ever be the target of such harsh life-destroying energy. Like Dr. Timothy Brown says, use this as mantra when frustration rises and you want to blame someone.

No blame.
No shame.

Enter the mind of an experienced gardener. Check out the condition, and you will surely discover a problem with the condition. Fix this condition, and the people will take care of themselves.

The world is made up of two things—the things that we want and the things that we don't want. When we appreciate something, the thing that we appreciate *appreciates* in *value and amount* in our lives. When you appreciate fine clothing, you will value them more and you will end up having more of those same fine clothing in your closet. By looking at what people value and gather, you can tell what they truly appreciate. Therefore, ponder on the things that you want.

Never have thoughts that are displeasing, but rather those that are *pleasing* to you. Your feelings should *not* be those of what you hate, but *what you love*. Your words should *not* be words of confusion, but *words of clarity*.

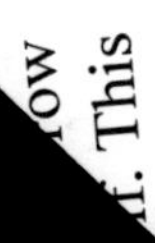

The misunderstood story of cholesterol

It is common knowledge that cholesterol is bad. But is this true? Let's examine what cholesterol is all about, in order to dispel this terrible myth.

First, only animals make cholesterol, so plants cannot produce it. In biochemistry, I learned that cholesterol's primary function is to stabilize the *cell membrane*. You see in plants or fungi that another layer called the cell wall protects the fragile cell membrane. However, the animal cells do *not* have cell walls. If they did, animals would not be able to move flexibly.

I sometimes see margarine manufacturers coming up with ways to sell more of their *hydrogenated* products. They claim, "Zero Cholesterol."

The claim is true, but misleading. They are riding on the concept that cholesterol is bad, and their unspoken subtext is that their product is good because it doesn't have any cholesterol in it. Of course, they fail to disclaim that cholesterol is *not supposed to be* in products made from plants in the first place.

However, a little research will reveal the dangers of margarine due to the presence of hydrogenated oils, also known as the trans fatty acids. Already more than 12 years ago, there were convincing data that show the dangers of hydrogenated oils. Transfats, such as margarine raised Lp(a), pronounced as "LP little A."[20] Elevated Lp(a) levels are associated with an increased risk of developing a heart attack, stroke or Alzheimer's disease. Studies show that while transfats raise Lp(a), saturated fats such as butter actually lowers it. So it appears that even butter is actually less harmful than margarine.

To sum it up, cholesterol isn't bad at all. On the other hand, what was considered good and healthy, the hydrogenated fat, and marketed as the healthy substitute for butter, is actually dangerous to your health.

Why is cholesterol considered so unhealthy? One of the functions of cholesterol is acting as a "rubber patch." When your car tire gets a puncture and begins to leak air, the mechanic would put a rubber patch inside the tire, and then re-inflate it. After the "patch job," the tire is as good as new. I have seen this work done on my own vehicle, and it is truly marvelous.

When your artery gets a tear and begins to leak blood, the liver will send LDL (low density lipoprotein) cholesterol to the artery. It will patch up the tear and hold the tear in place, so that healing can take place.

When the healing is complete, the cholesterol is removed from the tear, and it is returned back to the liver in the form of HDL (high density lipoprotein) for disposal. One main cause of arterial tearing has been recognized as lack of vitamins B6, B9 and B12. A lack of these vitamins converts an amino acid, methionine, into a toxic substance called *homocysteine*. Homocysteine causes the inner linings of the arteries to tear, which attracts platelets and LDL cholesterol to "patch up" the tears, and leads to hardening of the artery. This hardening can be measured by arterial stiffness index.[21]

A person living on fast foods and processed foods will often suffer a lack of B6, B9 and B12, which can cause continuous homocysteine injuries to the arteries, leading to many depositions of LDL cholesterol.

And here is probably *the one and the only one reason* why cholesterol is popularly considered dangerous. Massive cholesterol depositions that accumulated over time in the arteries can become loose and break off! This is known as *embolism*[22].

The *embolus* (the broken off piece of cholesterol mass) gets lodged (called embolism) in the brain causes a stroke. If it gets lodged in the heart artery, it causes a heart attack. If the cholesterol patch is lodged in the lumbar arteries, it cuts off the blood circulation to the discs and results in chronic back trouble and leads to disc herniation. If it lodges in penile arteries, it causes erectile dysfunction.[23]

The rise in LDL is *an indicator* of trouble in the artery, rather than a problem in itself. It is a sign of trouble, not trouble itself. It is easy to blame the LDL cholesterol for all of our troubles, and thus the widespread use of cholesterol-lowering drugs.

It should be noted that the cholesterol-lowering drugs do *not* heal the arteries. They merely delay the stroke or heart attack. You are supposed to find the root cause of the rise in cholesterol, and then remove the cause. The solution often lies in returning to eating wholesome foods, performing daily exercises, and reducing the body fat.

A side effect of cholesterol deposition in arteries is a rise in blood pressure. Over time, cholesterol can accumulate as more arterial injures are made that exceeds the rate of their healing. They form structures called *plaques* that narrow the lumen (the opening inside the artery through which the blood travels) of the artery. The result is increased blood pressure—just as you would get higher water pressure when you squeeze a garden hose when you water the plants.[24]

Blood pressure medications are often used for this condition, but again, they are *not* the cures. Of course, in all fairness, these medications *are* valuable because they will buy you *time* to change your lifestyle.

Blood pressure medications work primarily through reducing the blood volume. For example, thiazide water pills make you lose blood volume, and therefore, blood pressure.

Another way is to weaken the heart's contraction when it is pumping by blocking the heart muscle cell receptors with beta-blockers, such as atenolol. Depending on the dosage, the heart will pump with much less vigor.

One could also *numb* the arterial muscles from contracting by using calcium channel blockers such as felodipine.

Yet another way is using the ACE inhibitors, such as ramipril. ACE inhibitors were first isolated from the viper venom, which contained this poison. This poison paralyzed the arterial muscles, thereby disabling arterial muscle contraction. This results in a lowered blood pressure.

They are all effective methods, and when blood pressure is raging uncontrollably high, you must lower the blood pressure first, or the pressure can burst the artery, causing serious complications. But know that these therapies function only to *buy* some time. It is wise to, first, put out the "fire" and find out the solution to the problem.

Why it is harmful to blindly lower cholesterol

Cholesterol is one of the most important molecules in animal life. Cholesterol gives stability to the cell membrane, so that your cells don't crack or burst under temperature fluctuations such as when you go into a hot sauna, or jump into a freezing lake during the Polar Bear Swim on the New Year's Day. But there are more reasons why cholesterol is vitally indispensable.

All of your sex hormones, including testosterone, estrogen, and progesterone, are directly made from cholesterol. Without testosterone, one would not have any masculine qualities—such as your muscles, mental assertiveness, or motivation for action. Testosterone is known to heal your muscles after a workout, allowing your muscles to work out more frequently and heal more quickly.

Estrogen gives you the female qualities including breast development. Without it, all women would look like a prepubescent girl without the physical maturity of a woman.

Progesterone is a powerful mood enhancer. When a woman lacks it, she often feels depressed and easily irritated.

When athletes begin taking cholesterol-lowering drugs, one major side effect is the long-lasting DOMS (delayed onset muscle soreness). They report that the DOMS can last for weeks after an intense workout, instead of the typical one day or two. This is because cholesterol-lowering drugs inevitably also lower testosterone production.

Cholesterol is formed into bile in the liver, which is an emulsifier ("soap") that breaks large masses of fat into smaller fat droplets so that digestive enzymes can get to them and digest them down to the fatty acid units. Digestion of a fatty meal becomes difficult without bile and, of course, the body can suffer nutritional deficiency of a whole class of nutrients called *fat-soluble nutrients*. These include omega 3 fats and vitamins A, D, E, and K. A lack of omega-3 fats leads to systemic *inflammation*.

A lack of vitamin A is the number one cause of childhood blindness in Africa.

A lack of vitamin D is known to cause all immune problems (from allergy, cold, flu and cancer) to bone diseases (such as osteoporosis).

A lack of vitamin E contributes to free radical oxygen damage to the brain and nerve cells.

A lack of vitamin K leads to bleeding disorders.

When someone lacks bile to break down fat in the gut, the stool turns white in extreme cases. White stools are sometimes seen in patients who have undergone cholecystectomy—the gall bladder removal surgery.

The gall bladder normally receives bile from the liver, and stores it until it receives the signal from the small intestine. When the proper signal comes, the gall bladder releases the bile into the small intestine.

The briefly mentioned vitamin D is an essential fat-soluble nutrient. Without it, your immune system falls apart, and you become susceptible to more infections, more allergies, and puts you at a greater risk of cancer. Recent studies support the theory that this *sunshine vitamin* is crucial in cancer prevention[25,26].

So how is this sunshine vitamin linked to cholesterol? Cholesterol is found in all cells, including the cells lying in your skin. To put it simply, when sunshine (specifically the ultraviolet B radiation) strikes cholesterol in your skin cells, they vibrate and change their shape to become pre-vitamin D. They are absorbed into the blood stream, and get to the liver where they are processed by the liver's enzymes, and then reenter the blood stream to reach the kidneys where they become the active form of vitamin D.

As you can expect, when the cholesterol level plummets due to the use of cholesterol-lowering drugs, so does your vitamin D level. What follow are your immune problems.

The most popular drugs for lowering cholesterol, such as Lipitor, work by poisoning a key enzyme in your system. This enzyme is known as *HMG-CoA reductase*. This enzyme converts fatty molecules into cholesterol. The liver's ability to make cholesterol is reduced to the corresponding degree of poisoning. The more poisoning of the enzyme, the less the enzyme can make cholesterol. This, in turn, leads to corresponding levels of decrease in all the hormones made from cholesterol—testosterone, estrogen, progesterone, DHEA and vitamin D just to name a few.

Recent studies show that when HMG-CoA reductase is blocked, another crucial molecule found in the human cells is produced in less amounts. It is a molecule located in the inner membrane of mitochondria. This molecule is called coQ-10 (pronounced "ko-kyu-ten").

Without coQ-10, mitochondria cannot make the life-sustaining energy currency of all animals—ATP. ATP is the molecule of energy. ATP is used for *all* chemical reactions that occur in the body. No life is possible without ATP.

When the HMG-CoA reductase is poisoned, there is a significant reduction in the production of CoQ-10, which disrupts every mitochondrion's ability to produce ATP. Then the cells starve for energy, and in turn the person starves for energy. One becomes lethargic, and fails to grow, repair or reproduce—to the degree of the poisoning.

One simply cannot expect to maintain health while poisoning the crucial enzymes in the body.

There is yet another indispensable substance made from cholesterol. This is cortisol. Cortisol is released from the adrenal gland with at least two well-known functions: (1) to raise the blood sugar for the brain, (2) to calm down the naturally occurring inflammation in the body. Cortisol can also provide the "calm" that after an "adrenal rush" causes you to become overexcited and anxious. The lack of cortisol leads to a hyper-inflammatory state, and it can lead to symptoms of high inflammatory states such as pain, irritability, anxiety, itchiness and allergy.

As you can see, it is a widespread practice to use powerful pharmaceuticals to delay health tragedies, such as stroke and heart attack. However, one must proactively put some energy and time to resolve the underlying causes. When you simply engage blindly in treating the symptoms, and confuse the *markers* for the *disease*, complications will surely arise. High cholesterol is not the disease. It is a marker that there is a problem. Resolving the cause is the best way to resolve the symptoms.

The misunderstood story of osteoporosis

Here is another example of how the remarkable ability of the body to heal is viewed as an *engineering malfunction* in some dire need of correction.

The bones contain two crucial types of cells—osteoblasts [*osteon* Gk "bone"; *blastos* Gk for "to form"] and osteoclasts [*osteon* Gk "bone"; *klastos* Gk "broken"].

In other words, osteoblasts are the cells that form bones, and osteoclasts are cells that break down the bones.

Here is a philosophical question that you may be asking yourself when you realize that the body has both *bone builders* and *bone breakers*.

Question: Why does the body harbor and feed the osteoclasts that break down the bone? Is it a case of the body being infinitely stupid, or we just don't understand the process well enough?

Of course, the body is mysterious and there are numerous things that science does not understand yet.

Let's look at the nature of healthy bone maintenance. Let's say that you live in a twenty-eight-story high-rise condominium. After a mild earthquake, someone notices that there is a large crack that has appeared on one side of the building. The condo owners are understandably concerned, and the expert engineer is called in for the assessment of the damage.

The engineer assesses that a substantial repair is needed. The tenants have to be evacuated, the crack has to be torn out, and new support materials must be used to enforce the structure. It will take three months and costs $500,000. It's time-consuming and costly because you have to tear down the weakened parts before rebuilding it all to its previous structural integrity.

A dishonest builder comes around and says that he could fix that same crack in three days for $10,000. His solution was much *easier*. He will just fill in the crack with cement and put some paint over the crack. His solution requires no tearing down of anything. The cash-strapped strata council hears this and loves this idea. It's cheaper, faster, and requires no extensive repair than the first proposal.

If you were the strata president, which service would you choose? Isn't the proper way of doing things really the *only* choice? Unfortunately, when it comes to bone health, most people would rather choose the *easy way out* that could lead to some major problems in the long run.

Imagine that your bone gets injured with an excessive pressure on it—let's say from running a marathon, or jumping off a tipping ladder. Tiny fractures invisible to the naked eye form in the bones. You have both osteoclasts and osteoblasts. Which would you use? You can use the osteoblasts to fill in the fractured regions of the bone for a quick fix. But a wise choice is to tear out the fractured regions and lay down the bone thoroughly. Popular drugs called *bisphosphonates* are widely used to treat osteoporosis. An example of these drugs is Fosamax.

Bisphosphonate drugs cause a condition called Dead Jaw,

also known as the ONJ (Osteonecrosis of Jaw). It refers to a disfiguring condition where the bone *dies* and will not heal. In other words, once the jaw is broken in the Dead Jaw patients, the bone tissue fails to heal. This condition only occurs in people who have been on bisphosphonate drugs such as Fosamax and Actonel, Zometa, and Aredia, but never seen in any other groups of patients.[27]

The examples of LDL and HDL, osteoclasts, and osteoblasts are not the only misunderstood mechanisms that occur all the time in our body that keeps us functioning and breathing.

A car needs *the gas pedal* so that you can make the car move. But there should also be *the brake pedal* to make it stop when you need it to stop. Only when the two polarities exist, proper function can be expected. The opposing polarities exist throughout the body to keep it functioning at its peak potential.

Such polarity exists in the essential fatty acids. There are the inflammatory omega 6 fatty acids, and there are the anti-inflammatory omega 3 fatty acids.

The immune system has the inflammatory complement 6 and the anti-inflammatory complement 10.

In the locally acting paracrine hormones, there is the inflammatory PGE 2 and 4, and the anti-inflammatory PGE 1 and 3.

In the distant-acting endocrine hormones there is the testosterone that increases the masculine qualities, and the estrogens that increase the feminine qualities.

Also, there is the calcitonin that tells the bones to be built, and the parathyroid hormone that tells the bones to be broken down.

A thriving body requires a restraint of power of one polarity. Therefore, the harmonious interplay between the opposing forces is possible. A good control of the body's system requires more than the "gas pedal," but also the ability to "brake."

The body strives to maintain its set homeostasis to improve the chances of survival of the organism—your survival depends on the balance of the polarities. You cannot simply employ powerful drugs to shift the balance of power without eventually having to deal with the negative consequences.

Like any intelligent system, your body demands respect

The rule is straightforward: never *force* an intelligent system to reverse its actions, unless you clearly understand the consequences.

It is easy to block what the body is trying to do by using drugs.

There is a serious problem with the approach of forcing on the body the powerful anti-inflammatory drugs when it is infected with a flu virus. With the use of NSAIDs (non-steroidal anti-inflammatory drugs), a child can develop Reye syndrome, a lethal liver disease, and the child can die.

There is a problem when the primary treatment of a patient's osteoarthritis is the NSAIDs. NSAIDs merely attempt to force the body's inflammatory processes to stop. NSAIDs will remove the inflammation by removing blood from the joints. The pain of arthritis is the body's way of *informing* the patient to slow down activities long enough to give the body a chance to heal. Eventually, continued vigorous activities lead the arthritic joint to further break down, causing irreversible damage to the cartilage.[28]

As diseases deeply root, effective treatments become more invasive

Wisdom says, "Do not kill the messenger." It is an attempt to distinguish the message from the messenger. Similar advice would be useful in the healing fields.

The disease and the person need to be clearly distinguished. A skillful doctor carves out the disease without harming the person. However, when the disease is so *intertwined* with the person that it becomes nearly impossible to separate the two. This intertwining of person and disease leads to greater mortality due to procedures and treatments.

Mortality due to *preventable medical errors* in the American hospitals, is the *sixth leading cause of death*,[29] but it is *not* reported as such. The reason is that the CDC (Centers for Disease Control and Prevention) simply does *not* include this category in its annual National Vital Statistics. Nonetheless, it causes *98,000* deaths each year, and they are purely due to medical errors, and therefore totally preventable.

The accumulated knowledge in all the healing arts combined is not complete. Therefore, this must be clear: the treatment of choice should be the *least harmful* of all the possible choices for the patient, and it should be *the most reversible* of the possible choices just in case the procedure does not work.

Your potential life span is 150 years

You have the potential to live to 150 years old—without any further breakthrough technologies in gerontology. Let me tell you something fascinating that I learned in my biochemistry classes. In the mid-90s, we learned that a cell had a *clock.* A cell knew exactly how many generations it had descended from its ancestral fetal cell line called zygote. It is like you knowing how many generations of grandparents there were before you, and knowing how many generations there will be after you. I almost couldn't believe it, but it is a fact.

The most well known researcher in the study of aging is Dr. Leonard Hayflick. He published his research in 1961 from the Wistar Institute in Philadelphia, a biomedical center for cancer research. He discovered that cells would divide again and again, up to fifty times, and then they would stop dividing and die. The cells do not forever divide, but come to an end at a certain point. Hayflick discovered that a fetal cell line could go through cell divisions generation after generation up to fifty times.

Here is the mechanism that this author learned during schooling. With each cell division, the chromosome length shortens, and after fifty divisions, the chromosome reaches a critical length (having lost too many genes), stops dividing, and enters into what's known as the programmed cell death (also known as apoptosis). The limit of a cell's ability to divide is fifty times, and this limit is known as the *Hayflick's limit.*

With an average cell replicating *every three years*, you have 3 x 50 = 150 years as the *theoretical lifespan* of a human being.

Of course, that is, if you do it *right*. It is always possible to get into lethal accidents and contract various life-threatening diseases before your body even uses up the potential fifty replications.

The lifespan of 150 years is your *potential* and not your birthright. For instance, your favorite hockey team *can* win the NHL's Stanley Cup. But the Stanley Cup isn't a birthright to a team. It is earned through impeccable planning, lots of hard work, and perhaps some luck along the way.

I would like you to fully grasp the excitement contained in this chapter. You have the *potential* to live to a *healthy* 150 years of life, not 75 or 80. So if you are 75 years old, you better start planning the *exciting things* you want to do in the next half of your life—with your life experience and your cultivated wisdom.

Most of us are born with a great constitution for health

You have a great body that is meant to be reliable. Your body is able to heal enormous variety of ailments. However, there are problems that overwhelm your body's ability to heal. When you cannot heal on your own, you must seek medical help. There are largely two general types of therapies available—the first type is *supportive,* and the second type is *suppressive*.

When you have the flu and you provide the body with the needed rest and nutrition, you are engaged in a supportive therapy.

Supportive therapies do not contradict what the body tries to do, but rather work *with* the body. Supportive therapies would use remedies to allow the body to do what it needs to do in order to complete the healing process.

Contrarily, *suppressive* therapies tend to take over the healing process and override the body's tendencies. When the temperature rises, suppressive therapies would force the body to cool down. When arthritic pain rises, the suppressive therapies would use drugs to reduce the pain. Suppressive therapy simply tries to undo what the body tries to do.

Both types are valuable and can be used effectively for different purposes. Controlling therapies shine when the body is not able to mount an effective healing effort for a condition—either because the disease is too overpowering or the person has weakened too much. On the other hand, supporting therapies are perfectly fine when the body is still strong or the offending disease is not overpowering the person.

When you are shopping around for your health care professional, put some effort into your visit by being very clear in your mind about what health condition you would like to have resolved, and what your chief medical concern is. Fax or email any blood work or reports at least a day before seeing your doctor. No doctor will ever say that was such a terrible idea. It will make a doctor's job much easier to support you in your healing journey if you provide all the pertinent information.

Find a doctor who knows your health condition well

Although you are a healer, you still need the right conditions to heal. That is why you need a doctor. A good one.

Some patients live quite some distançe away. They invariably ask if there is a doctor that I can recommend. I gave this some thought over time. Everything being equal, a good doctor is mainly a keen observer, who would deeply contemplate your condition to guide you to the cure.

And no doctor can have mastered *all* healing arts. The more we learn, the more humble we become. Confidence is good in a doctor, but hubris is dangerous, as it is a symptom of ignorance.

The Mountain Climber[30]

An accountant dreamed of retiring as a farmer. When he retired, he bought an acre of farm, in which there was a cute house, a silo, and a well. He went and got himself a hen to get fresh eggs. He knew his farm well. One day he decided to climb the mountain behind his farm. He got up early in the morning and packed up his sandwich and water. Then he began climbing. After some time, he decided to rest on the flat surface of a rock. From there, he could clearly see the patch of land that included his own farm and 9 other farms. A thought entered his mind. "I see 10 farms so clearly, but I only know one of these 10 farms. My knowledge of this land is 1 out of 10, or 10%."

He began climbing again, and decided to rest after a few hours of vigorous climbing. When he looked down from the mountain, he counted 100 farms. A thought entered his mind. "I see 100 farms so clearly, but I only know one of these 100 farms. My knowledge of this land is 1 out of 100, or 1%."

He began climbing again, and reached the tippy top. He looked around and could clearly see farms reaching out as far as his eyes could see. He began counting, and he realized there were at least 1,000 farms. A thought entered his mind. "I know that there are at least 1,000 farms. My knowledge of this land is 1 out of 1,000, or 0.1%"

The old accountant saw a paradoxical trend. The more he saw, the less he knew. He concluded, "If I could see infinity, I would know nothing, as knowing 1 out of infinity, according to the exact science of mathematics is zero."

The universe was gentle enough to show him the limitations of knowledge. He understood in his heart for the very first time why Socrates, a man of great wisdom, claimed that he knew nothing.

Each doctor has a certain area of mastery. Find out what they have mastered, so that your condition has the greatest likelihood of healing completely. You don't have to rely on one doctor for everything. Spend some time to discover who is good at treating various conditions. Since a doctor cannot become an expert in every condition, it is wise to seek out different doctors for different conditions.

Focus on things that a few things that truly matter

It is the primary role of the physician,
Whether the African witch doctor
Or the modern doctor,
To entertain the patient
While secretly waiting
For nature to heal the disease.
Albert Schweitzer[31]

There is a common quality amongst great experts. They grasp the essential *principles* and then apply them in varying situations that they encounter on their daily situations. They think through problems, and make quick but surprisingly prudent decisions that bear positive outcomes. Once one has a good grasp of the principle, and the problem that one has encountered, the solution is merely in the application of the principles. Understanding the principles grounds the person in the state of certainty.

True experts do not necessarily use up their mental resources memorizing all the data; they simply commit to memory only the most crucial few pieces of information that really matter. This is also known as the Pareto's Rule of 80-20.

Pareto's Rule states that 80% of the effect comes from 20% of causes. Vilfredo Pareto, an Italian economist had noted in 1906 that 80% of land in Italy was owned by 20% of the population. He also noted that 20% of pea pods in his garden contained 80% of the peas. There are further examples, which include 80% of global wealth is owned by 20% of population[32]; 80% of sales come from 20% of product; 80% of shoes one wears are 20% of all the shoes one owns; 80% tax is collected from 20% of the population. The expert—the one who has honed one's skills to mastery—focuses on the 20% of the data that leads to 80% of the solution.

Similar pattern occurs amongst patients who do well in health. I have summarized these healing patterns below in three basic principles. Practicing the three principles can yield surprisingly a good result.

Some you may find the information below startling or even disagreeable. But I assure you that I have done the research that you should at the least keep these three principles in the back of your mind in the pursuit of your health. Here, are those important principles that you can use to build your health.

Nutrients are the building blocks of your body

Here, is the first principle of health—you are made up of nutrients.

People are mystified by the word, nutrition. I have heard of someone making a comment, "I don't believe in nutrition." It shows the depth of ignorance that pervades through our world as to what nutrition is all about. Nutrition is a major pillar of health. Simply speaking, nutrients are *the building blocks* for your body.

If one is building a house, one would require the tools and building blocks to do it. It makes no difference whether a person believes in the project or not—you need the necessary things. The fundamentals between building a strong body and building a strong house are still the same.

Every part of your body is ultimately made up of living cells. Cells then are made up of macromolecules—such as proteins, fats and carbohydrates. These macromolecules are further made up of nutrients. Nutrient categories are divided into seven categories—amino acids, fatty acids, simple sugars, vitamins, minerals and water. Our cells build all the necessary structures for itself and for the body, from the most basic building blocks called nutrients.

Nutrients are the basic units of one's body—the building blocks for the cells, tissues and organs, just like you would use building blocks (such as bricks, rebars, water, cement, windows, doors and nails) in constructing a building. This is why a fetus may fail to grow or may develop birth defects (for instance, spina bifida) when certain nutrients are lacking. A major cause of infertility in women is the *celiac disease*, where the small intestine become injured and cannot absorb adequate amounts of nutrients because of allergy to wheat, rye, and barley. In celiac patients, unless care is taken, there aren't enough vital nutrients to support the growth of the fetus in the mother's womb. A woman can successfully become pregnant when the needed nutrients become available in adequate amounts in the body, such as when the celiac disease is resolved.

A lack of nutrients will also halt the body's repair process. Repair processes in your body can be impaired when some of the nutrients needed for the repair are missing. That would delay both the healing and overcoming of diseases.

This author would like to view nutrients as the *letters of the alphabet*. The main building blocks for writing a book are the letters of the alphabet. If I am missing even one of the twenty-six letters of the alphabet—let's say I don't have the letter "A"—I would find completing this book to be impossible. Realistically, I couldn't even write my name without the letter "A."

Eating the Small COW diet

What is a *Small COW Diet*? It stands for eating *small* portion meals, made of *Cooked*, *Organic* foods chosen from a *Wide variety* of plant sources. The *Small COW Diet* is an ideal diet. I say this because it is relatively free of a number of dangerous substances. These include—environmental toxins, naturally occurring plant toxins, artificial sweeteners or flavorings, and pesticides. The Small COW diet also provides the high amounts of antioxidants, and the high concentration of vitamins and minerals per serving.

People often ask me why I recommend that their foods be *cooked*. They become a little startled by my suggestion. Didn't our ancestors eat raw fiber in nature-with dirt and germs and all?

Sure, eating raw foods has its advantages. Some nutrients are heat-sensitive, and the cooking process can destroy them.

However, unless you have a doctor or a health expert who is very familiar with the raw food diet and is actively guiding you to eat raw foods for a *specific purpose*, avoid this diet.

Instead, practice eating cooked foods as a general rule. Here is why I recommend against eating raw foods for a sustained period of time. It's because of the *toxins*.

Toxins in plants?

Yes, exactly.

Most plants contain naturally occurring toxins that are eliminated through the *cooking process*. These naturally occurring toxins include psoralens, phytates, trypsin inhibitors and solanine alkaloids. These can wreak havoc in your health. These are, in fact, plants' natural biological pesticides to protect themselves. Fortunately these toxins are heat-sensitive and can be destroyed through the cooking process.

Let us examine some of these toxins.

Psoralens cause your skin to become photosensitive, and when psoralens in your skin are exposed to the sun's ultraviolet radiation, they become photocarcinogens. Photocarcinogens are cancer-causing agents when the person is exposed to the sun's rays. Psoralen-containing plants include celery, parsley and parsnips. A few grams here and there are perfectly fine. However, you do not want to juice them and consume them daily in large quantities.

Phytates are especially abundant in soybeans and other legumes. Phytates are also in nearly all whole grains, and most berries. These plants must be cooked thoroughly to destroy the phytates. Phytates are *anti-nutrients.* They bind up *minerals* in the gut and get them eliminated as stool so that you develop mineral-deficiency. Because berries and nuts are not generally cooked before eating, avoid *excessive* consumption of them, such as relying on them for sole caloric intake.

Whole foods, not processed or refined, are truly the best for building a healthy body. The reason is obvious: simply stated, the whole foods contain all the original nutrients that they are supposed to contain—amino acids, simple sugars, fatty acids, vitamins, minerals, fiber, and water. The moment they are refined, they begin to lose some of the vital nutrients. Sugar cane has all of the above nutrients in varying amounts, but the refined sugar has only sugar. Once refined, the sugar cane product now lacks amino acids, fatty acids, vitamins, minerals, fiber and water. The sugar provides calories, but they lack any other essential nutrients. That is why they are called *empty calorie foods*.

Due to the increased transportation distance of food since the industrial revolution, the shelf life of various foods has become a key economic problem. The wholesalers do not want their foods to be spoiled before reaching the market. Therefore, they looked for ways to increase the shelf life of their produce. One good example is the successful prolonging of the shelf life of flour.

When the grain is ground, the fatty acids in the germ layer become exposed to oxygen, and become rancid in about six months. Since a general understanding of fatty acids and vitamins was lacking in the 1800s, removing the germ was an excellent solution. "Degermination" was a technological and an economic triumph, but it was also a public health failure. Degermination was a triumph because the white flour had a much longer shelf life, and it could be preserved for years for the lean times as well as for the long distance transportation to reach the target market. But it was also a failure, as rare diseases began cropping up. These diseases include the below:

Vitamin B1 is known as thiamine. B1 deficiency is called *beriberi*. Vitamin B1 is involved in breaking down glucose for energy. A deficiency can cause extreme lethargy, heart failure, and possibly eventual death. It is called *Korsakoff's syndrome* if the B1 deficiency occurs in *alcoholics*.

B2 is also known as riboflavin. It is what is making someone's urine brightly fluorescent yellow after taking a B-complex pill. The B2 deficiency is especially a concern for a young couple expecting to become pregnant. It's because B2 deficiency leads to such conditions as *cleft palate* deformity, growth retardation of limbs[33] and congenital heart defects.[34] It can be avoided by avoiding excessive consumption of refined foods, which are often devoid of these essential B vitamins. Also, ruling out celiac disease that prevents nutrients from being absorbed is crucial. There are simple lab test that tests you for celiac disease.

B3 or niacin deficiency leads to the infamous *3Ds of pellagra*—dermatitis, diarrhea and dementia.

B6 or pyridoxine deficiency leads to seizures in infants, anemia in adults, and heart disease. This may be due to the rise in homocysteine.

B9 also known as folic acid deficiency leads to anemia, neural tube defects in fetuses that cause *spina bifida*, and heart disease through the rise in homocysteine.

B12 methylcobalamin deficiency leads to anemia, peripheral nerve damage, and damage to the white matter of the central nervous system. Again, B12 deficiency is yet another B vitamin that is linked to heart diseases.

You see the importance of avoiding refined foods, and return to eating whole foods. But also eat the whole foods grown organically to avoid chemical pesticides. The heating process, unlike the biological pesticides, cannot destroy chemical pesticides.

Further exploration into plant toxins

Most plants have some toxins. Plants have developed more than 10,000 natural compounds that protect them against threats to their existence.[35] Currently, there are less than 1 percent of all plants that have ever lived on Earth, and this tiny percentage of all the plants survived partially because of their toxicity.

The toxicity of aconite is well known. A bean-sized aconite seed can kill a person. Here are some others: azalea causes coma. Black nightshade, or petty morel, especially the unripened fruit and leaves, causes hallucination and paralysis[36]. The watery juice of castor oil bean contains powerful toxin called *ricin* which is lethal (but the oil is absolutely harmless). Daffodils cause blurry vision or death. Deadly nightshade, or greater morel causes muscle paralysis and death. Foxglove causes irregular heartbeat. Hemlock causes death. Strychnine kills through muscle convulsion in about three hours.[37]

If you check the Government of Canada website on "Poisonous Plants information system[38]" you will realize that some of your favorite fruits and vegetables are also listed—alfalfa, aloe, avocado, buckwheat, croton, garlic, mango, oats, onion, cherries (various types), potato, radish, rhubarb, St. John's wort, sunflower and sweet pea.

So why isn't everyone violently ill from all those plants?

The answer is simple. Our ancestors experimented with them, and taught us to process them in ways that reduced the toxicity—such as baking, frying, fermenting and steaming.

The intention for this section so far was not to scare people of foods. Neither was it to ask people to eat a narrow list of foods. In fact, the intent is to appeal to one's logic, and establish an understanding of how to eat foods in a safer way. It is *unwise* to pick and select a few items of food and consume only those. In fact, that would be the worst thing to do.

Harmful substances are present in nearly all plants and meats[39] in varying amounts, and the toxic effect increases exponentially with the increase in the amount. One does not want to "load up" so to speak on one toxin. The toxic effect is reduced significantly when each type of toxin introduced into your body is small in quantity. So instead of picking and choosing from a few types of plants, do exactly the opposite by selecting a *wide variety of food.* Only then can you minimize the toxicity. Incidentally, the practice of eating a wide variety increases the likelihood of you consuming the full-range of essential nutrients. The following are the various toxins that you should be aware of to maintain your health.[40,41]

Aflatoxins: They come from the mold that grows on peanuts, corn, wheat and rice—those that are grown or stored in moldy conditions. Aflatoxins cause liver damage and liver cancer.

Anti-vitamins: Antivitamin-A—found in whole grain rice, it can cause blindness if enough of the antivitamin-A binds up all the available vitamin A in the bloodstream. Although vitamin A deficiency is rare in Canada and the US, it is nonetheless a common problem in Africa. In fact, vitamin A deficiency is the *leading cause* of blindness in African children. Antivitamin-B1 toxin is present in mung beans, rice bran, beets, Brussels sprouts. By cooking them, you destroy this toxin. Antivitamin-biotin (anti-B7) called avidin is present in raw egg white.[42] By cooking the egg white, you destroy avidin.

Amylase inhibitors: The enzyme amylase is an important starch-digesting enzyme present in saliva and the small intestine. Wheat contains a group of anti-enzymes that inhibit amylase. Cooking destroys this toxin. However, you should realize that this toxin is still found in the less cooked areas such as in the center of the bread.[43]

Cyanide is a powerful toxin from plants that warns animals not to eat their seeds and their young. They are abundant in the *seeds* of many common fruits such as apples, grapes, and apricots. Cyanides are also found in lima beans and young bamboo shoots. Cyanides are mostly absent in the flesh of fruits. They cause respiratory distress and mental confusion. Large amounts are lethal.

Amygdalins: Apples, pears, apricots and peaches contain a naturally occurring substance, *amygdalin*. Amygdalin turns into cyanide in the stomach and can cause discomfort or illness. Apricot kernels should be limited to a maximum of two kernels per day. Tapioca is processed from cassava. Cassava and bamboo shoots also contain cyanogenic glycosides that are broken down into cyanide in the stomach. They must be cooked thoroughly to destroy the toxins.

Goitrogens: Goitrogens are also known as the glucosinolates. They are present mostly in brassica[44] (also known as cruciferous vegetables) family such as cabbage, broccoli, cauliflower, canola, rapeseed, Brussels sprouts, kale, turnips, mustard seeds, and horseradish. Goitrogens cause hypothyroidism by making iodine in food unavailable to the thyroid gland. Since the thyroid hormones raise the metabolism of all cells in the body, the effects of goitrogens are lethargy and weight gain—consistent with typical hypothyroidism due to other causes.

Hemagglutinins are present in mostly uncooked legumes. Hemagglutinins retard the growth of a child.

Nitrates and nitrites are contained in celery, lettuce, spinach and cabbage. Nitrates and nitrites are also artificially added to cured meats to kill germs that spoil meats. Nitrates and nitrites decrease the oxygen-carrying ability of red blood cells in infants, causing anemia-like symptoms. With decreased levels of oxygen, the infants fail to thrive. Nitrates and nitrites also cause colic in infants, and they are the known cause of stomach cancer in adults.

Pyrrolizidine alkaloids include solanine in the "greening" potatoes and tomatoes. They cause vomiting, diarrhea and severe headaches.

Lathyrogens are in *legumes* such as chickpeas and sweet peas. When legumes are relied on as the major source of calories in the diet, the lathyrogens act as *glutamate neurotransmitter-antagonists*, and cause crippling *paralysis* of lower limbs along with osteoporosis. Lathyrogens may cause death.[45,46,47] You must always cook legumes *thoroughly*.

Furocoumarins: Parsnip contains furocoumarins. Furocoumarins accumulate in great concentrations in parsnips when the parsnip plant is *distressed* from insect bites or weather changes. Concentration is highest in the peel. Fucocoumarin toxins cause painful stomachaches and painful skin reactions when the person is exposed to UV rays at the same time.

Glycoalkaloids: Potato's glycoalkaloids (including solanine and chaconine) inhibit cholinesterase, and cause an abnormally long half-life of the neurotransmitter *acetylcholine*. Anti-cholinesterase toxicity symptoms include GI (gastrointestinal) upset, but also rapid and difficult respiration and even death. The common *pesticides* organophosphate insecticides are anticholinesterase as well, and cause a similar toxicity picture. Glycoalkaloids are low in normal potatoes, but higher in potato *sprouts* and the *peel*. They will taste *bitter* when the toxin concentration rises. Stress from insect bites, bruising, and UV exposure increase the toxin production. Deaths have been reported overseas, but they are extremely rare.

Lectins: Kidney beans contain lectins, causing GI upset, but most importantly, lectins are agonists (has similar properties) to insulin. Therefore, lectins bind to insulin receptors, and cause *disruption in blood sugar* metabolism—such as *hypoglycemia* and *weight gain*.[48] Cooking destroys the lectins.

Trypsin inhibitors: Soybeans contain an abundance of trypsin inhibitors that interfere with protein digestion. Cooking and fermenting destroy the soybean toxins. Miso is a popular Asian food that has been prepared by cooking and fermenting, which make them safe to consume in larger amounts.

Oxalic acid: Rhubarb contains oxalic acid, and in high concentrations it causes muscle cramps and decreased muscle and heart functions, and even leads to coma.

Man-made toxins: Avoid man-made toxins. These include coffee, trans fats, artificial sweeteners and pesticides. *Avoid these toxins as much as possible*. This should be fairly straightforward. But humans are not so rational. Would you allow your precious children to drink coffee and eat donuts all day, then allow them to smoke cigarettes and drink alcohol all night? Probably not. Then why would you ever do that to yourself, unless you do not wish health? You are as precious as any child—at least to yourself and your loved ones. Do your best to remove toxins from your body. Sweat them out, or chelate them out, but get rid of them and make sure you don't take them into your body to the amounts that interfere with health.

The habit of careless uptake of toxins into the body may seem harmless now, but they eventually can cause problems. You don't pay for them now because the harmful effects are like that of folding a piece of paper that initially starts slowly, but grows in thickness exponentially, or the story of the penny doubling every day that adds to millions of dollars within a month. Initially, it seems innocuous enough, but very quickly the effect of various toxins can become insurmountable.

Eating well

Do not think in terms of "nuts are good," "berries are the best," "brown rice is the way of eating healthy," and so on. They are all good, and in proper portions, and in small amounts, they will give you the best anti-aging effects.

Practice eating the *Small COW Diet*—small portion meals made of Cooked, wholesome Organic foods picked from a Wide variety of plant sources. We have a tremendously good warning system built-in to our body. It is called the *gut upset*. Your gut will tell you if you are eating something that you should be avoiding.

Your gut is really a long tube of hollow muscles. When it gets irritated, it means that it has detected something that could be harmful for the whole body. It *does* the one thing it knows how to do—it goes into a muscular spasm. This is why you might feel nauseated when you unwittingly ingested irritants. Irritants in your food tube may even cause vomiting (a violent food tube spasm) if the food hasn't passed the stomach. Diarrhea would result (violent intestinal spasm) if the irritants have already passed the stomach.

If you get GI symptoms, find out which food is responsible, and cut it out from your diet for *three days* before reintroducing it in normal proportions. As a general rule, never eat moldy nuts and grains. Cut out the green spots on potatoes and tomatoes before eating.

Humanity began cooking 1.9 million years ago

Dr. Chris Organ found evidence that human ancestors were outliers amongst other primates in one major way—*the chew time*. Dr. Organ examined the animal's percent of the day spent on chewing from studying the tooth sizes and body masses of the modern humans, the human ancestors, chimpanzees and other modern apes[49].

The human ancestors generally spent less than 10% of their day chewing. The modern humans spent 4.7% of the day chewing. Homo erectus (lived 1.9 million years ago) spent 6.1% of the day chewing, and homo neanderthalensis spent 7% of the day chewing. Homo habilis (lived 2 million years ago) spent 7.2% of the day chewing.

In comparison, the modern chimpanzees chew 48% of their days. The reduction in chewing time is due to cooking. Cooking allowed greater extraction of calories from food. Since the brain is extremely calorie hungry, being able to extract greater amounts of calories allowed for greater brain development and greater intelligence.

The biological anthropologist, and the author of *Catching Fire: How Cooking Made Us Human*, Dr. Richard Wrangham[50], a former student of Jane Goodall in 1970s makes similar suggestion. Wrangham says that cooking made tough fibrous plants and meat parts more digestible, increasing the caloric extraction and decreasing time invested in finding and chewing food. Cooking would have also killed off many harmful germs present in foods, as well as the toxins present in many species of plants to a safer level. Cooking thereby reduced the morbidity and mortality in human ancestors to make them one of the most successful procreators of all time.

Our ancestors were not carnivores, herbivores nor omnivores. Humans are meant to be consumers of *cooked foods*. Cooking is why humans have out-competed other ape species and left such numerous progeny to this date.

Consume cooked whole organic foods. Understand the limitations of nutrition—that they are the building blocks. Taking less than the needed amounts of nutrients will make you not thrive. Taking more than you need, and you will not benefit any more than taking the needed amount. Avoid refined foods. Avoid restaurant foods—unless they can cook like you would at home.

The circulatory system and the lymphatic system

Reading is to the mind what exercise is to the body."
— Joseph Addison

We have two main fluids in our body. The first is the circulatory system that contains the blood. The second is the lymphatic system that contains the lymph. When people hear statements like, "Body is 60 percent water," they immediately think that the body is *60 percent blood*—which would be forty-five liters of blood for a 165-pound person. However, that is incorrect. In reality, we only have about five liters of blood, accounting for a mere 7 percent of our body. So where is the rest of the water?

Much of the water is within the cells, of course. Another large portion is in the lymphatic system. Your lymphatic system is roughly *three times* that of your blood system. The lymphatic system's function is to *bathe* all the cells in your body. It is the lymphatic system that supplies the cells with nutrients, so that your cells can perform their life-sustaining chemical reactions. It makes enzymes, hormones, neurotransmitters, nonessential nutrients, and so on.

When you *move* your lymphatic system, you are actively pumping out stagnant fluids around the cells that contain mostly waste products such as—ammonium and carbon dioxide. At the same time, the movement of lymph fluids encourages nutrients to enter the cells.

Improving the delivery of nutrients into cells through muscle contraction

Exercise and application produce
order in our affairs, health of body, cheerfulness of mind,
and these make us precious to our friends.
Thomas Jefferson

Everyone should exercise. Exercise provides your body with many important benefits. First, exercise causes muscles to go through a series of contractions and relaxations. This muscular action causes the old lymph fluids to be pumped out the tissue and allow the new lymph fluids to nourish the tissue cells.

Question: While the *heart* pumps the *blood*, what pumps the *lymph fluid*?

To find the answer, we should look at *exercise*. Exercise means you are moving your *muscles*. As you move your muscles, the contracting muscles put a "squeezing" pressure on the lymphatic system, and it is this muscular contraction that causes lymph to start moving. In other words, the force of muscle contractions pumps the lymph fluids.

This is why a massage feels so good, beyond what the resulting muscle relaxation can provide. The lymph system is well designed in that it has veins with backflow-preventing valves that allow the lymph to move in one direction only, sequentially moving the fluid toward the heart, and eventually draining it into the blood.

Another benefit of exercise is that it makes you look good. Your skin cells are nourished through exercising. Let me elaborate on that. Your largest organ is your skin. I got that question wrong in one of my exams because I thought of an organ as something within the body, and I had not thought about the "covering." The skin is about 15 percent of your total body weight. If you are 150 pounds, you have 23 pounds of skin.

Under normal circumstances, the skin rarely gets nutrients. So how do you get the nutrients to nourish the skin? The best way to get some nutrients into the skin is by activating the sweating mechanism. Sweating occurs when the body temperature rises sufficiently high to trigger the natural thermoregulation mechanism in hypothalamus, and cause the tiny blood vessels in the skin to open up. This lets out the *water* and the *electrolyte* portion of the blood, thereby releasing heat with it. This is the trick to skin rejuvenation. When you exercise, your skin will get nourished as a side effect.

The third benefit of exercising is the body's hormone regulation. Our bodies are really gigantic *pharmaceutical* factories. They can produce any hormones and neurotransmitters that you need—let that be testosterone, estrogen, growth hormone, endorphin and serotonin, just to name a few.

However, our hormone/neurotransmitter-producing glands only produce them when they receive the correct signal. The signal is your lifestyle. Your lifestyle determines what hormones and neurotransmitters your body will produce. Our bodies are adapted to survive various seasons. In the abundant summer season, our ancestors ate frequently and moved much. Anthropologists agree that our ancestors forty thousand years ago walked *fifteen kilometers* per day looking for food, interspersed with rapid sprinting and tree climbing when they ran into predators. This is not too far from the ideal way to keep your own body fit and muscular. Brisk walking daily, interspersed with intense exertion, results in good muscular tone, healthy bone density, and strong ligaments.

A number of well-done papers looking at marathon running indicate that marathon running is associated with heart damage, and the risk is highest with those who are less fit[51]. Dr. Eric Larose studied the effects of marathon running on heart using MRI and VO2 max tests before and after marathon running. He reported that marathon damages the hearts of less fit runners for up to three months[52].

Exercise does not mean that one needs to run marathons. It simply means to challenge the body enough to keep the muscle and bone mass. The quality of fitness-inducing exercise program is defined not by the length, but rather by the intensity. Dr. Martin Gibala at McMaster University discovered in his studies that a short-term intense training that consisted of only six repeats of 30 seconds of high intensity exercise was equivalent to lengthy 90-120 minute endurance training in enhancing the fitness level[53]. The body can be in a great physical shape doing only a few minutes exercise per day three times a week.

Exercising the power of faith

We can all learn from the common stamp.
It sticks to the envelope until it reaches the destination.
Abraham Lincoln.

Faith is inner vision multiplied by inner conviction

Although faith and belief are often synonyms, here I will define the two differently. Belief is believing in something external. You may have a belief in someone's promise, a philosophy or a religion. A belief often influences our thought patterns and behavioral patterns.

While I define belief as something external having an internal manifestation; faith is an internal force that has external manifestation.

The first component of faith is the inner vision

Inner vision is distinguished from what the two naked eyes see. Our eyes can see a distance. It may see 500 meters. Or with an aid of a powerful telescope, it may be able to make out people's faces 10 km away. When the telescope lenses provide high resolution under the correct light condition, it can see very far. However, the vision is still in the realm of distance—and it cannot cross the boundary between distance and time.

In order to see into the future, one has to activate the inner vision. In the spiritual circles, they call this the 3rd Eye. Because it is in the realm of the 6th sense, one needs to quiet down the five senses in order to access it.

With practice, one is able to magnify the resolution in viewing the future. You would notice that the future is not set yet. The possibilities are many—from the best scenario to the worst scenario, and everything expected and unexpected in between two extremes. The inner vision allows us to "see" into the future, and "nail down" the future that you desire. The inner vision gives you the goal—or target.

The second component of faith is the inner conviction

Inner conviction is your ability to stay committed to the goal that you have set out. Once you have the target, you should finish it, and then reassess the action in entirety. We all have heard the story of the miller and the donkey. Below is a synopsis of the story.

The miller, his son and the donkey

A miller with his young son took the donkey to the market to purchase some flour. The two walked happily alongside the donkey. It wasn't more than a few minutes had passed when they ran into a passerby who commented how stupid they were to have a strong donkey and not use it to carry one of them.

The father and the son thought about it and realized the passerby made sense. He put his young son on the donkey, and began walking when another passerby stopped them. He commented that it wasn't good that a young healthy boy would let his aging father to walk under the hot sun while the boy rides comfortably on a donkey.

They saw the logic, so they switched. Now the father is riding the donkey while the son walked beside him. It wasn't more than a few minutes had passed when they ran into another passerby who stopped them. He commented how uncaring it was for a father to let his young son to walk under the hot sun while the father himself rides comfortably on a donkey.

They realized that he had a point also. So the father and the son both got on the donkey. It wasn't more than a few minutes had passed when they ran into another passerby who stopped them. He commented how abusive the father and the son were to make the donkey carry both of them under the hot sun. They realized that this passerby made sense also.

Running out of options, the father and the son decided to carry the donkey.

Once you have seen the various possible futures, and you have nailed down the one that you desire, you need to stay strong to stay on-course. The moment you have made a decision, the universe tests your resolve by bringing to you circumstances and situations that pushes and pulls you off the path you walk—just like the passerby's who make comments to the miller and the son. This is why one needs inner conviction. Having inner conviction allows you to stay on-course. Imagine you are a spy in one of the major Hollywood spy movies, where the spy shoots an arrow with a rope attached, and then *zip lines* all the way to the target. The wind may try to blow you away off course, but the spy makes a rapid progress towards the target.

The persistent focus of a cat

I had a cat that I thought was cute, but I never thought of it as a wise teacher. One day, I woke up in the middle of the night to go to the bathroom, and I saw my cat sitting in the kitchen. He was intently focused on something but I didn't know what. He barely acknowledged me as I passed by. That was quite unusual. He sat in the kitchen day and night, and from the looks of his bowl, he barely ate. I would have taken him to a vet, except I noticed he wasn't ill. The cat was focused on something behind the kitchen drawers. His focus was so intense that I decided to one day see what he was up to.

He wouldn't move from one particular area and I truly became curious, but also a little worried. Eventually, I had to bring his food tray and water closer to him so that he might eat. Even then, he rarely ate or drank. Then on the third day, around 2:00 am, I heard a tremendous fuss in the kitchen, and when I went and checked it out, I found my cat triumphantly looking at me with a tiny *mouse* in its mouth. I swear I think I saw the cat smiling. It was the first time I saw a cat with a mouse between his teeth.

I grabbed the cat, and took him to the lawn outside. I pried open his mouth, and the mouse fell out—rigid like a piece of twig. I thought the mouse died. After all, a cat's teeth are sharp. Just to check if the mouse was all right, I used a piece of stick that I could find to give it a nudge. To my surprise, the mouse bolted right up, and took off. I think it may have recovered from a fainting spell, and found its opportunity to escape. I am glad that it did. My cat struggled to be freed, determined that it won't let its prize getaway. I grabbed my cat with both arms and took him inside.

Trying to look away from my cat's blaming eyes after I let his prize go into the bushes, I tried to rinse my cat's mouth—just in case the mouse was infected with any pathogens. Then, I sat on the sofa and thought of the times when I was *as obsessed* as my cat catching the mouse. Faith is at work when one sees his higher vision and persistently walks the path with a sense of a deep inner conviction. Upon exercising his faith repeatedly, he begins to see the glimpses of the unchanging laws in operation all around him. This is when he comes to a sense of inner certainty.

Fear paralyzes

Courage is not action in the absence of fear,
but in spite of fear.

Fear's purpose is to paralyze you in times of uncertainty. It therefore, buys you time. When you have more time, you can generate more options. From a larger pool of options, you can make better choices.

When you don't know what to do, inaction until getting to better know the environment can mean the difference between a success and a disaster.

However, there are times when you know that an action is beneficial, but you are paralyzed simply because your emotional muscles have atrophied through a lack of use. For those moments, practice on a daily basis, doing the things that you know are good and wise. This will strengthen the emotional muscles and boost the mental horsepower.

Do first what you fear the most. See how this changes your perception of the world. When we pass on from this world, most of us would be more regretful of the inaction than the mistakes we made.

When a person constantly grows, one also constantly enters into the world of the unknown. Growth simply means that one has entered a new height where one has not reached before. A growing person is bound to *make mistakes* as the new territory is previously an undiscovered territory.

May you have the courage to overcome your fears. May you have the courage to enter into the new heights of your awareness where embarrassing mistakes are possible, but also where the most delicious nectars of life are abundant. No one great has earned admiration for having remained in safety.

Have fewer thoughts

Of all the countless thoughts that we have each day, how many of those thoughts are truly our own? Our minds are bombarded with snippets of thoughts from TV commercials, clever advertisements, chitchats, and news articles. Universe was gentle enough to send me to a temple in Taiwan to spent four months in a Buddhist temple as a monk, and I found something that I had not known before.

The monks spent much of their time working on a very few, but very high-quality thoughts. Their thought vibrations were so high, that I found their behaviors constantly resonating with, for the lack of words, *virtue*. Here, I use the virtue to mean the highest levels of conduct. It made sense to me. The highest levels of thoughts led to highest levels of conduct.

They taught me to avoid "thinking many thoughts," but rather "think fewer thoughts." This gave me a different understanding of being thoughtful. "Being thoughtful" to the monks meant the depth of quality, not breadth of quantity.

With fewer thoughts to work on, the mind becomes a capable tool, excavating each thought intensely. Only then, do we have the capacity to mull over our assumptions carefully, remove the chaff and fluff from our paradigms as we reflect them upon our conscience.

What these monks gave up in variety, they were rewarded in intensity. The mind, like a magnifying glass, only has power when there is the intensity, not variety. It is in the intensity that a thought becomes a workable plan, and the workable plan becomes a brilliant strategy that inspires a series of constructive thoughts and actions. Then those thoughts and actions lead to the corresponding physical manifestation.

Your empowering vision keeps you focused

A powerful vision is the lighthouse that keeps you on course and gives you hope in times of darkness. For the best possible outcome, formulate an empowering vision, a clear identity of self, and knowledge of a big payoff when the goal is manifested.

A *vision* is a declaration to the universe. You are stating to the universe where you wish to go. When you give birth to a worthwhile vision, it will contain a power of its own. Its power will pull you through even in the most challenging of times.

A clear *identity* tells the world who *you* are. A lack of self-identity manifests itself in hypothetical thoughts and goals that are time wasting, as this lack the anchor of self-knowing. As the great thinker, Socrates once said, "Know thyself." Know your strengths, weaknesses, visions and values—then live your life of contributing to the world in a way only you can.

A solid *game plan* is your strategy for manifesting the vision. A solid action with power requires certainty of your mental resolve. A powerful mental resolve arises from a solid game plan that you believe will work. Spend time focused on mapping out how you will get to your vision. Be the pioneer and explorer of your own life. In the end, it is infinitely more powerful to have a game plan than no game plan at all, even if that game plan is an awful one. An awful game plan can be modified once you are in action, as the feedback of trial and error will ultimately guide you toward the best way to reach your goal once you are in motion.

Brief Reflection on Maps

by Miroslav Holub

Albert Szent-Györgyi[54], who knew a thing or two about maps,
By which life moves somewhere or other,
Used to tell this story from the war,
Through which history moves somewhere or other.
From a small Hungarian unit in the Alps a young lieutenant
Sent out a scouting party into the icy wastes.
At once
It began to snow, it snowed for two days and the party
Did not return. The lieutenant was in distress: he had sent
His men to their deaths.
On the third day, however, the scouting party was back.
Where had they been? How did they manage to find their way?
Yes, the man explained, we certainly thought we were
Lost and awaited our end. When suddenly one of our lot
Found a map in his pocket. We felt reassured.
We made a bivouac, waited for the snow to stop, and then with the map
Found the right direction.
And here we are.
The lieutenant asked to see that remarkable map in order to
Study it. It wasn't a map of the Alps
But the Pyrenees.

There is a greater chance of reaching the target by action than by inactivity. Even if the plan may not be perfect, a plan nonetheless is more productive than not having a plan. A plan, even if it is a wrong plan, puts you in charge of your life.

Two Brothers

The older brother was blessed with wealth, but had no family. The younger brother was blessed with a large family, with a beautiful wife and six healthy kids, but always had trouble with not having enough food for the family.

Lying in bed one night, the older brother thought, "My younger brother has six kids to feed, and he can barely make ends meet. I should secretly go and carry a bushel of grains from my silo and add it into my younger brother's silo at night after everyone has fallen asleep."

Lying in bed the same night, the younger brother thought, "My older brother is not blessed with family. At least he should enjoy wealth." The younger brother decided to deliver secretly a bushel of grains from his silo and pour it into his brother's silo early in the morning before anyone was awake.

The next morning each brother was puzzled to see that his silo had as much grain as the day before. Each one thought, "I can share more with my brother." So they did exactly the same thing that night. The older brother secretly delivered a bushel of grains very late at night; the younger one delivered grain very early in the morning. But again, the next morning, each brother was puzzled to see that his silo had as much grain as the day before. Each decided that he could share more again. This continued on for five days.

Then one day, under a full moon, the older brother started out later than usual; the younger one started earlier than usual. They ran into each other in the middle of the path by the hill where they used to play as kids. Finding a bushel of grain on each other's backs, they realized what had been happening. They have been trading grains secretly every night! They both became tearful at how much they cared about each other.

Each brother had a need. The older one didn't have a family. The younger one didn't have much wealth. But they didn't focus on their own needs, but on what they could serve the other. Heaven on Earth is created when people focus on expressing their love without an expectation of love in return. That is a world of peace, joy and grandeur. May we all stop "calling for love" and start "expressing love." A Course in Miracles would say that this occurs when the fear-based thinking has grown into love-based thinking.

Quality of life through the depth of love

As one becomes a lover,
Duties change to inspirations.
Practices become dance...
Coleman Barks[55]

"Who loved me and who did I love?" According to Elizabeth Kubler-Ross, this is the question that people ask themselves in the last hours of their lives. The dying person would scan through the memories from then, all the way through as far as they could remember, and try to recall who loved them and who they loved. When they cannot find such examples of love, they would become depressed.

There are two questions that the dying people ask—who loved them, and who they loved. In analyzing the two questions, we realize that the second question is much more powerful than the first question. "Who loved me" has everything to do with other people. We know that no matter what we do, being loved depends on the willingness of others to love us. However, loving other people has everything to do with us. We can choose to love someone unconditionally. That is why it is a much more powerful question. If we are going to ask these questions at the last hours of our lives, we should start working on them right away when there is still some time.

Life is meant to be fun. Observe children when they are playing. They show so much happiness and creativity, it makes you smile. It doesn't take much to be happy and joyous. Even our physiology is designed to have fun. The mood-enhancing chemicals are much stronger than any exogenous morphine. And the body naturally produces them. These are known as endorphins. Also present in the human body are the endocannabinoids, the happy chemicals made by the body, thought to be responsible for the "runner's high." Endocannabinoids include anandamide [Skt *ananda* = "delight"] and 2-AG (arachidonoylglycerol).

Happiness is not *there*. It is *here*. It is not to be pursued, but practiced. It is here within everyone's grasp. You are a blessed person if you can write down ten things that make you happy right now. Think of the memory of your baby's first smile. Return to those moments when you spent joyous times with your loved ones. Think of remembrance of you overcoming your various fears. Think of you doing something that you thought you couldn't do. We tend to forget these things because once we reach a new level of achievement, we forget how far we have come, and begin seeking something even greater. We tend to forget to acknowledge the distance we have traveled so far. Sit down before moving on to the next segment of your life. Mentally acknowledge just how far you have come to arrive at this point. Celebrate your greatness. Only then, move on.

The world is filled with great things to learn from. Be a constant learner so that you can continue to expand your awareness. Even committing a crime may need awareness according to history. Queen Min[56] asks the crown prince which is a worse crime—a crime committed knowingly or unknowingly. The crown prince replies that it is the crime committed knowingly that is worse because the crime had been committed twice—once in mind and once in action. The Queen replies, "That is why you are not the king yet."

The Queen says that a criminal who commits a crime unknowingly will commit the crime again and again until he becomes aware that he is committing a crime. On the other hand, a knowingly committed crime begins to attack the conscience of the criminal during the quiet of the night when there is no one else around. It is in the quiet of the night, the criminal has to face himself in full honesty. The criminal who knows of his crime is more likely to repent and later, atone through acts of kindness to others when his conditions improve. The lesson to the crown prince was that a wise king has to think differently from the people he takes care of, and that he must continue to study; even a criminal has to understand why he is doing what he is doing.

Evolution of human consciousness

As mentioned previously, I was taught the three qualities of a mature being—wisdom, compassion and courage. I forgot about the three virtues through my late teens. Then, in my twenties, I began having nightmares.

In my dreams, I would act very foolishly. It caused chaos in my life and everyone else's. I would get up in the middle of the night from the nightmare, feeling really bad about my actions in my dreams.

Another night I would dream about being the pettiest, the most unloving person who lives a very cold, emotionally isolated life because I have no compassion for others. I would then wake up from the dream and the trauma of the event. Another night, I would dream about being a coward, a true coward who betrayed his loved ones because he couldn't stand up to the heat.

Each time I would get up around 3:00 a.m., and I just could not go back to sleep. I was ashamed of how I thought and behaved in my dream. Dreams often show us a side of ourselves that is unconscious. In "real" life, if I have a tendency to behave a certain way that I do not approve of, I would override that with more appropriate behavior. But in the dream world, I seem to be *naked*. I behave the way I feel, and that feeling gets exaggerated several times over. If I am sad in my dreams, I am endlessly sad. If I am happy, I become also polarized in that passion.

That was what was bothering me. I would ask myself, "Am I really foolish, selfish, and cowardly as in my dreams?" But what bothered me the most was that it was all a dream! In a dream, I could do anything. I could have tested out my wisdom. I could be as generous and compassionate as I wanted—or as courageous I desired. I could risk my life for a great cause, and the price I paid really would be just waking up from the dream.

A dream can provide a safe place to express your wildest imagination. You can be as grand as you wish without paying the price. It is like having a movie with you as the superhero that is all wise, compassionate and courageous. However, in the dreams, I missed these opportunities, and I would be up at 3:00 in the morning saying I must get back to my dreams so I can correct them.

An awakening

An epiphany occurred: the dreams are not real, but they did really and truly feel real. I used to dream of ghosts, and they were very scary. Sad dreams were just too sad. Happy dreams are so energizing that I would start flying in my dreams. In fact, at times, I would run so fast, I could step on air molecules and climb up into the sky!

A dream is an illusion, and I know it is an illusion *when I wake up*. A dream is a place that I visit for a few hours every night, and then I wake up from it. My waking up tells me that the dream was an illusion.

New resolution

Dreams can feel more real than reality itself. Perhaps the

dreams are there to remind us that our reality is simply another dream from which we awaken after 80 years of slumber. When we awaken from the 80 years of slumber, we may ask ourselves, "Was I wise?" "Was I compassionate?" "Was I courageous?"

Saibaba once said that "I - ego = God." From self, if we removed our ego, what is left is God. I am not certain that we can completely be free of ego. In fact, I am not even sure if it is a good idea to eradicate ego while living on Earth. Ego does provide a reference point for our being. Life on Earth is a temporary thing. Time flies by, and towards the end, we get to ask what this life was all about.

I have observed that a great life is made up of great actions. Great actions are beyond the simple functions of the ego. Also, I know that when people truly care for a cause, they act free of ego. You see this in the battlefields, as well as in friendships. One thinks big to do big things. One's life is too precious to live small.

Enlightenment in a coin

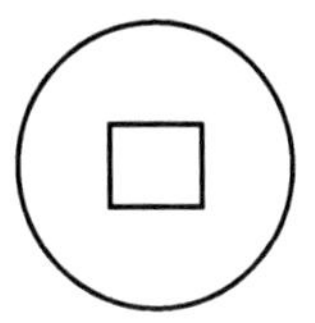

You can reach enlightenment meditating on an ancient coin. The ancient coins used in many Oriental civilizations were round with a square hole punched out of the center. These coins not only were valuable as money, but also for their philosophy.

Growing in Korea, I heard phrases such as "Inside Square, Outside Round." The sharp-angled square represents *stability*, like a boulder in a shape of a cube, while smoothly curving roundedness represents friction-free *movement* like the most perfectly polished pearl.

Your inner world should be sharply defined, with crystal clarity of your vision, values and awareness. The outside world should be rounded with its gentle curvature, as to not cause friction with the rest of the world. This person who has attained Inner Squaredness and Outer Roundedness has a powerful inner world of vision that guides the person's life, while maintaining a frictionless relationship with the outside world. This is considered ideal.

There are three other possible coins

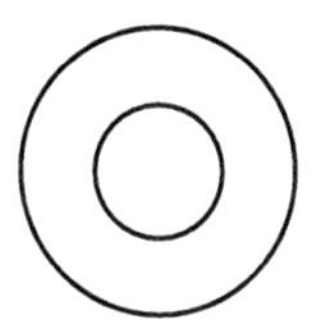

A person can be *Round Inside and Round Outside*. This person is ever so changing in his vision depending on the outside circumstances and situations because he has no real vision of his own to begin with. He never spends any time or energy developing his personal codes of conduct, or developing his empowering vision of the future he would like to create. This person has no *color* and therefore blends in with the others, and he never really gets anything meaningful accomplished because he lacks persistence. He is always dominated by the outside power.

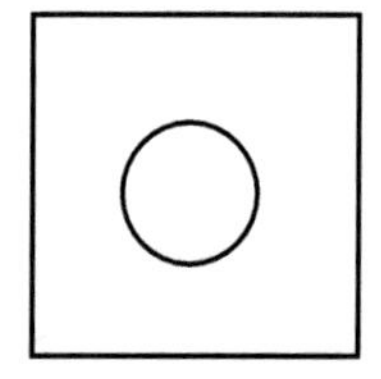

Another person can be *Round Inside and Square Outside*. This person is very difficult to get along with because of his character flaws. He seems to be attached to minor things for a majority of the time, and he lacks organization in his Inner World. He always gets into trouble with the world, and his "nose" gets bent out of shape on a daily basis for no apparent purpose other than getting his short-terms wishes met. He always seems to be pushing for an agenda, but that agenda has neither substance nor consistency. His Inner World is tormented because he has never experienced what it's like to have a stable, organized Inner World.

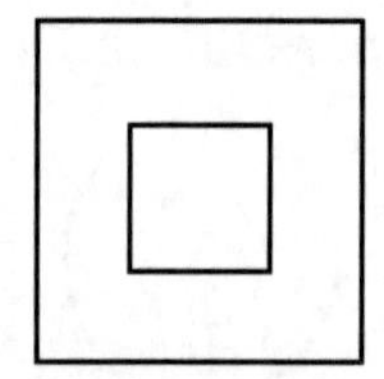

The last type is someone who is *Square Inside and Square Outside*. He usually cannot co-exist with the world, and he must live a life of a hermit. He has a strong conviction about an issue, and will push and push for it relentlessly, while being completely blind to the outside world. He may put some ideas together, organize a group of fanatics, push for a cause, and relentlessly pursue it. However, the world does not tolerate this person for too long, and this person is driven to live in isolation.

Three mindsets of human awareness

A person is born dependent. He uses resources up but is not able to contribute. He learns from the older ones, especially his parents, uncles, teachers, mentors, and finally becomes independent. An independent person continues to grow and begins to work with others who are independent. This leads to interdependence. The dependent, independent and interdependent stages can also be a physical stage, emotional/mental stage, and spiritual stage. A dependent person who fails to take the path toward independence may choose co-dependence as a means to survive. Such a person in this dependent stage forms a unit with another dependent person, not for the purpose of thriving, but for surviving.

The human spirit is truly endless.
Find the way to grow, and then persist through it.

I see a vision: small puddles in the ground gather a special type of water, called consciousness. Each puddle is not enough to support life, but it is born after a rainfall of life. Disconnected from one another, they have limited consciousness—and one day they will dry up and that would be the end of them. They wait for the rain of life to come, but some realize that with the rise in consciousness, they could raise the "water" and join with other puddles around, forming a pond, which can support life and longer sustenance, as the larger body does not dry up so easily. The further rise in consciousness finds rivers and underground water supplies to raise its consciousness; ponds, brooks and streams join in their consciousness to form lakes and rivers that can last thousands of years, and their petty differences are secondary to the bigger and powerful vision they dream together—to have a collective consciousness.

Four ways to overcome stress

Humans effectively overcome stresses through four means. These are science, arts, humor and faith.

Science objectifies the problem that is causing the stress. In the scientist's mind, he identifies the problem, and turns that into a project that can help others. It is the scientist amongst the primitive people who decided that putting a piece of animal skin on their feet could help them ease the foot pain from walking on a rough surface.

An artist would write a song or poem about the challenge, and discover a deep hidden meaning that makes the challenge worthwhile. Art is the axe that cracks the ice that reveals the noble heart beneath. It is the axe that shatters the darkness and brings in the light of consciousness.

Someone else would use humor to deal with stress. He recognizes the humor in a challenging situation. Most of all, he find humor in himself. One becomes capable of laughing at himself. The humor makes you laugh, and the stress then diminishes.

Another one way to overcome stress is faith. (Read the chapter on "Exercising the power of faith.") Faith is made up of two noble qualities called inner vision and inner conviction. Faith enables one to see beyond the five-sense reality, and thereby allow the breakthrough to become possible.

Imagine

Row, row, row your boat,
Gently down the stream.
Merrily, merrily, merrily, merrily,
Life is but a dream.

An American nursery rhyme

I have heard Dr. Wayne Dyer interpreting the above nursery rhyme.

According to Dr. Dyer, one should row one's own boat—and not try to row someone else's. It says that, one should row gently, not roughly or forcefully. The direction of the boat is down the stream, not upstream. The rowing is done with open delight and joy. The time we spend on Earth is only an ephemeral dream and will soon come to an end. At the end of life, we will be left with nothing but the memories of how we faced the events of our lives. In other words, it is all about our own reaction to the circumstances and situations. Since it is just a dream, you can be as brave and merry as you wish.

Like the nursery rhyme, at the end of life, many things that we fuss about now may turn out to be insignificant. When we realize that many things didn't matter that much at the end except for the warm love that we exchanged, the laughters that we shared and the growth that we experienced.

People may find that there is one key difference between a person who has found one's internal light and who has not. The difference is in how they love, laugh and grow. The *un-*

enlightened person needs a suffering to kick-start his growth. An *enlightened* person can grow through self-reflection, and has no need for suffering. Only the ones who remain in the dark require suffering as the sole vehicle for growth.

Self-reflection comes to us in the moments of *stillness*. *Profound insights* can only come during those prolonged periods of stillness that are free from the strains of lethargy and illness.

Imagine a life where *your body* is reliable and strong, and graceful to look at. Your life is not of pain, depression, fatigue or emptiness. Rather it is those of joy, optimism, vigor and purpose. This joyous state of being is what being healthy is all about. Only when one has truly mastered health, can one maintain the prolonged infusion of pure insight to accelerate your own evolution.

May you attain a reliable body, and maintain it. Once you get healing out of the way, you can begin exploring the other dimensions of life—filled with vigor, inspiration and joy.

Endnotes

1. ERdoctorpetpeeves.http://www.youtube.com/watch?v=mEDQItVCxbw&feature=related. Sep 13, 2011.
2. CNN Wire Staff. Motorcyclist's uncle tells nephew's rescuers, "You are heroes" September 13, 2011.

3. Nature here doesn't mean herbs or sunshine, or any other physical aspects of nature. Naturae should be defined in its original Latin term "*natura*" to mean *the inherent tendency* in something. Just as a red blood cell delivers oxygen or a muscle fiber contracts, a living thing heals. Natural contains the Latin *nat* (born) and *ura* (result). Nature indicates *the inborn tendency* of an entity. It explains how seasonal birds know where to migrate, how trees know how tall to grow, how the sun knows how bright to shine, and how the Earth know how fast to rotate. Therefore, the antonym of "nature" is *artificial* or *forced*, in the context used in this book.
4. The block of marble had a fatal flaw near the right foot. It prevented many artists include da Vinci from taking on the challenge. Michelangelo at 26 years of age saw not the flaw, but a tree stump that supported David's right leg.
5. As of 2009, cancer has surpassed heart disease as the number one cause of death in the U.S

6. Twombly, Renee. "Cancer Surpasses Heart Disease as Leading Cause of Death for All But the Very Elderly." *JNCI Journal of the National Cancer Institute* 2005 97(5):330-331; doi:10.1093/jnci/97.5.330 http://jnci.oxfordjournals.org/cgi/content/full/97/5/330
7. Heron, M; Hoyert; D, Murphy; S, Xu; J, Kockanek; K, Tajada-Vera, B. "Deaths: Final Data for 2006. Table B.

Percentage of total deaths." *National vital statistics reports*, vol. 57, No. 14, April 17, 2009

8. It's fascinating to realize that the third leading cause within the category of accidental death is due to conventional medical procedures
9. 2003 American Heart Association conference.
10. 25 years of age is a personal observation. It is observed that the body tends to heal much slower after the age of 25.
11. Noticeable pain reduction occurs usually only after the first treatment. Five treatments performed over 8 weeks tend to be the average number. The healing does depend on one's overall health, the therapist's skill level, and the patient compliance during the treatment period.
12. http://www.reliabilityindex.com/manufacturer
13. Cole Christopher, Blackstone EH, Pashkow FJ, Snader CE, Lauer MS. Heart-rate recovery immediately after exercise as a predictor of mortality. N Engl J Med 1999; 341:1351-7.
14. Of course, the figure 99 is a metaphor.
15. It is always amazing to see a paradox. The wealthiest parts of the town tend to have the cleanest houses and streets while the poorest neighborhoods tends to have the dirtiest houses and streets. It is a paradox because the wealthiest neighborhoods consists of the busiest people, and the poorest neighborhoods consists of the highest number of unemployed people. One would expect unemployed people to have more time on their hands to keep their neighborhood in tiptop shape.
16. Muscle also burns glucose, but it has its own storage, and will not access the glucose in blood under normal conditions. The exception is when the muscles have depleted their glucose storage, which (like the liver) store glucose in the form of glycogen.

17. Pablo, Carlito. "Shelter costs in Vancouver eat up income." *Georgia Straight*, March 6, 2008. http://www.straight.com/article-134790/shelter-costs-eat-up-income
18. Panzenboeck, E. "Housing Affordability in British Columbia." *Business Indicators*. September 2008. http://www.bcstats.gov.bc.ca/pubs/bcbi/bcbi0809.pdf
19. They worked very hard for these, and they are still working very hard to pay for the mortgage. Consider the origin of the word *mortgage*. People who speak a Romantic language would see the root, "mort," in the word, referring to death. Mortgage [*mort* = death; *gage* = solemn promise] is a solemn promise to repay the loan under the penalty of death. Mortgages, and borrowing money beyond one's limits, should be considered carefully.
20. Lichtenstein, AH et al. Effects of different forms of dietary hydrogenated fats on serum lipoprotein cholesterol levels. The New England Journal of Medicine, June 24, 1999.
21. G Vyssoulis, E Karpanou, S-M Kyvelou, D Adamopoulos T Gialernios, E Gymnopoulou, D Cokkinos, and C Stefanadis "Associations between plasma homocysteine levels, aortic stiffness and wave reflection in patients with arterial hypertension, isolated office hypertension and normotensive controls." *J Hum Hypertens*, 24(3): 183–189, March 2010.
22. By the way, people are often confused between thrombosis and embolism. Thrombosis is when blood clots slowly and gradually, and eventually blocking an artery. Embolism is a big piece of matter, usually cholesterol chunk, that gets lodged in an artery. For example, in a stroke is due to blockage of an artery that supplies blood to the brain. If one gets "thrombotic stoke" the onset of the stroke is slower than an "embolic stroke' where the onset is sudden.

23. Penis is a sophisticated balloon. Penile arteries inflate the penis causing erection, and later the veins remove the blood. If the arteries are blocked with cholesterol plaques, erection would be slow or impossible.
24. If you squeeze the tip of the garden hose, the same amount of water must travel through the narrower opening, and therefore pressure rises. You see this increased pressure by observing the greater distance that the water squirts out.
25. Lappe JM, Travers-Gustafson D, Davies KM, et al. Vitamin D and calcium supplementation reduces cancer risk: Results of a randomized trial. *American Journal of Clinical Nutrition* 2007; 85(6):1586–1591.
26. Wei MY, Garland CF, Gorham ED, et al. Vitamin D and prevention of colorectal adenoma: A meta-analysis. *Cancer Epidemiology, Biomarkers, and Prevention* 2008; 17(11):2958–2969.
27. Rubin, Rita. "Drug linked to death of jawbone." *USA TODAY,* March 13, 2005. http://www.usatoday.com/news/health/2005-03-13-jawbone-deaths_x.htm
28. However, you must also understand the complexity of arthritis such as rheumatoid arthritis. The degeneration is so fast that sometimes the most reasonable treatment is to use the most powerful anti-inflammatory drugs to slow down the permanent cartilage damage.
29. "HealthGrades Quality Study: Patient Safety in American Hospitals." *HealthGrades*, July 2004. http://www.healthgrades.com/media/english/pdf/hg_patient_safety_study_final.pdf
30. This is a story originally told to this author by a Vancouver philosopher, Hugh Atrill. With him, this author co-created a philosopher's club called "Discovery" and we spent over 10 years meeting every Friday at 7 pm. He was indeed one of the most brilliant persons this author has

ever met.

31. Dr. Schweitzer shared the same philosophy of Voltaire when it came to the role of a doctor.
32. Ross-Larson, Bruce et al. Global dimensions of human development. Human development reports published for the United Nations Development Programme, Oxford University Press. 1992. P. 35
33. Robitaille J, Carmichael SL, Shaw GM, et al. "Maternal nutrient intake and risks for transverse and longitudinal limb deficiencies." Data from *the National Birth Defects Prevention Study*, 1997-2003. "Birth Defects Res A Clin Mol Teratol." April 6, 2009;[Medline].
34. Smedts HP, Rakhshandehroo M, Verkleij-Hagoort AC, et al. "Maternal intake of fat, riboflavin and nicotinamide and the risk of having offspring with congenital heart defects." *Eur J Nutr*, 47(7):357-65, October 2008. [Medline].
35. Purdue University http://www.four-h.purdue.edu/foods/Naturally%20occuring%20toxins%20in%20foods.htm
36. Black nightshade poisoning. MedlinePlus. http://www.nlm.nih.gov/medlineplus/ency/article/002887.htm
37. en.wikipedia.org/wiki/List_of_poisonous_plants
38. http://www.cbif.gc.ca/pls/pp/poison
39. Meats contain even more dangerous toxins. These include Paylean or ractopamine. It increases disability in livestock, but used widely in US because it increases lean body weight of animals. Then there are the antibiotics, PCBs, dioxins, and abundance of saturated fats. On top of all this, meats contain many plant toxins that the animals had consumed.
40. http://www.healthy-eating-politics.com/toxins-in-food.html
41. New Zealand Food Safety Authority. http://www.nzfsa.govt.nz/consumers/chemicals-nutrients-additives-and-

toxins/natural-toxins/index.htm

42. Watson DH, Ed. "Natural Toxicants in Food. Progress and Prospects, Ellis Horwood Series." *Food Science and Toxicology.*
43. Watson DH, Ed. "Natural Toxicants in Food. Progress and Prospects, Ellis Horwood Series." *Food Science and Toxicology.*
44. Heaney Rk, Fenwick GR. "Natural toxins and protective factors in Brassica species, including rapeseed." *Natural Toxins,* 3(4):233-237, 1995.
45. Liener IE. "Implications of antinutritional components in soybean foods." *Critical Reviews in Food Science and Nutrition,* 34(1):31-67, 1994.
46. Heaney Rk, Fenwick GR. "Natural toxins and protective factors in Brassica species, including rapeseed." *Natural Toxins*, 3(4):233-237, 1995.
47. Seawright AA. "Directly toxic effects of plants chemicals which may occur in human and animals foods." *Natural Toxins*, 3:227-232, 1995.
48. Pedro Cuatrecasas and Guy P. E. Tell. Department of Medicine, and Department of Pharmacology and Experimental Therapeutics, The Johns Hopkins University School of Medicine, Baltimore, Maryland 21205Proc. "Insulin-Like Activity of Concanavalin A and Wheat Germ Agglutinin-Direct Interactions with Insulin Receptors (glucose transport/lipolysis/adenylate cyclase/affinity chromatography/lymphocyte transformation/growth factors)." *Nat. Acad. Sci. USA,* Vol. 70, No. 2, pp. 485-489, February 1973.
49. Man entered the kitchen 1.9 million years ago. Jennifer Welsh. Live Science, August 22, 2011. http://www.livescience.com/15688-man-cooking-homo-erectus.html
50. Gorman, Scientific American, January 2008, "Cooking up bigger brains."

51. Neilan TG et al. Myocardial injury and ventricular dysfunction related to training levels among non-elite participants in the Boston marathon. Circulation. 2006 Nov 28;114(22):2325-33.
52. Larose, Eric. Marathons damage the hearts of less fit runners for up to three months. Canadian Cardiovascular Congress 2010, Montreal. Oct 25, 2010.
53. Gibala et al. Short-term sprint interval versus traditional endurance training: similar initial adaptations in human skeletal muscle and exercise performance. J. Physiology pp 901-911. April 2006.
54. (September 16, 1893 – October 22, 1986) was a Hungarian physiologist who won the Nobel Prize in Physiology or Medicine in 1937. He is credited with discovering vitamin C and the components and reactions of the citric acid cycle.
55. Barks, Coleman. In his book, *Rumi, the Book of Love*. P. 38. Harper Collins.
56. Queen Min, also known as Empress Myeongseong (1851-1895) was the last queen of Korea.

CPSIA information can be obtained at www.ICGtesting.com
Printed in the USA
LVOW120003180712

290482LV00004B/3/P